BASIC EPIDEMIOLOGICAL METHODS AND BIOSTATISTICS

A Workbook

BASIC EPIDEMIOLOGICAL METHODS AND BIOSTATISTICS

A Workbook

Cecil Slome
*University of North Carolina
at Chapel Hill*
Donna R. Brogan
Emory University
Sandra J. Eyres
University of Washington
Wayne Lednar
*The Walter Reed Army Institute
of Research, Washington, D.C.*

Wadsworth Health Sciences Division
Monterey, California

Wadsworth Health Sciences Division
A Division of Wadsworth, Inc.

Printed in the United States of America
10 9 8 7 6 5 4 3 2 1

Library of Congress Cataloging in Publication Data
Main entry under title:

Basic epidemiological methods and biostatistics.

    Bibliography: p.
    Includes index.
    1. Epidemiology—Methodology. 2. Medical statistics. I. Slome, Cecil. [DNLM: 1. Biometry.
2. Epidemiologic methods. WA 950 B3115]
RA652.4.B38   610' .723   81-16278
ISBN 0-8185-0486-2   AACR2

Sponsoring Editor: *Edward F. Murphy*
Production Service: *Brian K. Williams*, San Francisco
Manuscript Editor: *Carol Westberg*
Interior Design: *Janet Wood*
Cover Design: *Al Burkhardt*
Illustrations: *Carl Brown*
Typesetting: *Graphic Typesetting Service*, Los Angeles
Production Service Coordinator: *Stacey C. Sawyer*
Design Coordinator: *Jamie Sue Brooks*

Dr. Cecil Slome died shortly before this manual went to press. We dedicate it to him in warm memory of his love for epidemiology and his strong desire that students learn it in a way that would maximize their interest in the field through minimizing tedium.

Preface

There are many viewpoints on *epidemiology*, but all serious definitions and descriptions confirm that it is a science concerned with the distribution of health, disease, and health behaviors in human populations. The Greek derivation of the name (*epi*, about or upon; *demos*, populace or people of districts; and *logos*, word, thus science or theory) indicates that the unit of study is not an individual, but a group or aggregate of individuals. Epidemiology is a science concerned not only with epidemic diseases, but with all health states in human populations. In addition, epidemiology comprises both a body of knowledge and a method. The epidemiology of one or more health states, therefore, is indicative of the state of knowledge surrounding the occurrence of the health states in human groups and the factors associated with them.

Epidemiological methods, as opposed to epidemiological knowledge, are a compilation of concepts and strategies derived from, and shared with, many related sciences but applied to the study of health and disease in populations. The basic strategy is one of comparing the health experiences of two or more populations in a way that produces a picture of the populations' health and explains any observed differences by developing and testing reasons or hypotheses.

As a community research tool, epidemiology can estimate how frequently a health event is distributed differently in some groups than in others. With this information, directed and logical steps can be taken to change appropriate aspects of the community so as to improve its level of health. Therefore, epidemiology is the diagnostic and evaluative science needed for objective and scientific community and public health practice.

Because of its application to health and disease, epidemiology turns for concepts and interpretations to other health sciences such as biology, medicine, genetics, dentistry, and microbiology. Similarly, its focus on groups rather than individuals requires the incorporation of methods and concepts from other sciences addressed to human groups and their functions. Hence, many indices, theories, and processes of human interactions are derived from sciences such as sociology, psychology, and demography.

Biostatistics, and its related mathematical bases, has a special place in epidemiology. It contributes ways of quantifying observed phenomena. Biostatistics permits the estimation of the likelihood of occurrence of health attributes under specified conditions. It also lends more scientific rigor and certainty in describing and analyzing epidemiological comparisons and associations and in deriving inferences from such analyses.

Because it is a science that concerns the health of humans, epidemiology generally uses an observational, rather than an experimental, approach to explain the health attributes of groups or aggregates of individuals. The observational mode is a limitation, as compared with laboratory-based research in which control and regulation of the factors of interest and the elimination of distracting factors are possible.

When possible and ethical, the *experimental* mode is indicated and used in epidemiology—for example, in testing new drugs or a new form of health care delivery. In such experimental epidemiological trials, however, certain ethical considerations and individuals' rights of informed consent, participation, and other freedoms of choice make the experimentation less controlled and rigorous than in the true laboratory-based study.

There are many experiments that, if performed, would provide more certain knowledge of causes of diseases in humans, but we would— or should—baulk at such experimentation. The observational approaches of epidemiology and related sciences are possible, with very selected experimental back-up. They are slower but very deliberate. Above all, because it usually is not based on experiments, but on observation of true human situations with all their variabilities, epidemiology addresses real-life situations—desirable property in a science addressed to humans.

Stallones accurately describes the *raison dêtre* of epidemiology:

> I believe that we have a central axiom, not subject to proof, but upon which epidemiology is based, and without which no epidemiology is possible.
>
> *Axiom:* Disease does not distribute randomly in human populations.
>
> *Corollary 1:* Nonrandom aggregations of human disease are manifested along axes of measurement of time, of space, of individual personal characteristics, and of certain community characteristics.
>
> *Corollary 2:* Variations in the frequency of human disease occur in response to variations in the intensity of exposure to etiologic agents or other more remote causes, or to variations in the susceptibility of individuals to the operation of those causes [Stallones RA: *Ann Rev Pub Health* 1:80, 1980].

This manual is addressed to the concepts, methods, and strategies of epidemiology. The learning of any substantive knowledge about health states, derived from the illustrative examples, is fortuitous. The manual does provide the initial and basic learning that is necessary to further epidemiological activity.

The manual is a guide for learning skills and concepts in a progressive manner. It begins with techniques of counting health events and ways to express their frequencies; continues with the strategies and methods used in carrying out a study; considers potential sources of weaknesses, strengths, and errors in those methods; and then pursues the conclusions that can and cannot be derived. This path of learning stresses ways of comparing health effects or outcomes in different populations, the rules of evidence needed for accepting observed differences, and the possible nature of associations found.

Finally, the manual guides you through the development of a study, presenting some thoughts that are necessary throughout. In a sense, this last section puts all the parts together.

Cecil Slome
Donna R. Brogan
Sandra J. Eyres
Wayne Lednar

How to Use This Manual

This manual will guide you in learning the basic concepts and principles of the scientific method, along with related biostatistics, that are used in epidemiology. Its format permits your learning in your own time and at your own speed. Some considerations in the manual may appear inordinately simple, but our experience and our students' experience suggest that a refresher on these basics is almost always of value.

Having a teacher available as a resource is a bonus but not a necessity for learning from this manual. Access to selected references will considerably enhance the benefit of working through it. A list of recommended and optional references is included at the end of each chapter.

Every chapter introduces one or more principles of epidemiology or biostatistics. Each exercise contains several thoughts and questions relevant to the concepts or principles, followed by comments.

In order to enjoy your learning the most, we recommend that you use the manual in the following manner. Do the chapters in the order in which they appear. Begin Chapter 1 with Exercise 1.1. After reading Exercise 1.1, stop, consider the thought or question, and write down your response to the exercise in the allotted space below the exercise. Then read and think about the Comment on 1.1, proceed to Exercise 1.2, and continue in the same manner. Writing your responses down in the spaces provided will promote your learning.

Throughout the manual, specific related references will be recommended. If possible, you should read these when you have completed the chapter, for they form part of the guided learning. Other optional references that extend beyond these chapters are included and can be pursued as you prefer.

At the end of each chapter is a summary of the concepts and principles covered therein. This will provide a review for you. If one or more of the concepts or principles are unclear, return to the chapter and review them before proceeding to the next chapter.

The manual also contains a glossary of terms for ease of reference and some optional self-evaluation questions. Answers and explanations to these questions are also given.

We have also included a descriptive bibliography of texts of epidemiology and biostatistics with our appraisals of them. We hope this list of currently available references is a help to you.

The manual is devised to facilitate your learning. It is good to recall that the "ledge" of "knowledge" is from the old English word meaning "play." Use the manual any time you are ready for learning, and not as an instrument of self-inflicted agony and memorization. We hope that your learning in this manner will be enjoyable as well as profitable, for then we will all move forward.

You may have differences of opinion with us on our thoughts; if that is so, then progress in your learning is assured. We would welcome your opinions, criticisms, or comments on this manual—they will assure our progress in learning.

In closing, we would like to thank the many students and colleagues too numerous to name who have helped in the development of this manual. We are indebted to them for their assistance.

Contents

Table Reading, Table Generation, and Rates: Some Epidemiological Essentials

1

As described in the introduction to this manual, epidemiology is concerned with the health and diseases of groups rather than of individuals. In order to pursue this endeavor and to describe the magnitude and frequency of occurrence of any health or disease event in groups, we turn to biostatistics for some tools.

A **rate** is a statistical way of expressing the proportion of people who have or develop a disease among all those in the total group who are at risk of having or developing the disease. Thus, a rate requires you to be able to say whether or not an individual in the group has or has not developed a particular disease or health outcome, and it attempts to summarize the group's experience into a simple expression.

Epidemiologists are said to play the numbers game. As you become involved in epidemiology, you will often need to present data in tables, which are little more than attempts to organize and present the meaning of numbers. So let us start right in with some tables.

Exercise 1.1

The numbers of Americans who died in selected years in the death registration states are shown in Table 1.1.

- ☐ Looking at the data in the table and using death as an indicator, do you think that Americans of 1970 are less healthy than their predecessors?
- ☐ What makes you think that?

Write down your answers in the space on the next page, then read the following discussion.

Table 1.1   **Total Deaths Registered, Death Registration**
States, USA, for Selected Years

Year	Deaths (in 1,000s)
1900	343
1920	1,118
1940	1,417
1960	1,711
1970	1,921

Source: *Vital Statistics of the United States, 1970.* vol. II, Mortality, part A, pp 1-2. US Department of Health, Education, and Welfare, United States Public Health Service, National Center for Health Statistics, 1974.

NOTE: In this and all other tables, you should *make sure that you read the headings.* Table headings are of great importance to understanding and interpreting data. This is an important basic principle in all table reading. A table heading should tell you the health outcome being measured (for example, death), the categories to be compared (years, age or sex groups, occupation groups, and so forth), the place where the group is located (for example, USA), the time or time interval (1900, 1960, 1940–1970, and so forth), and the index being used ("rate per 1,000," "means," or whatever). In short, the table heading should tell you the who, what, where, and when of the data.

Comment

Note immediately in Table 1.1:

1. These are data for the United States and only for death registration states. Hence, prior to 1933 they do not refer to the whole nation because all states were not yet included in the death registration sys-

tem. It is not essential for this chapter, but if you wish to pursue sources of health and mortality data, read references listed at the end of Chapter 1.

2. The data are for selected years. Showing years ending in zero is common in tables containing health information because these are the years of the decennial (every 10 years) US Census of Population and Housing.

3. The figures given are *numbers* of deaths registered.

4. These figures appear to be small because they are in thousands.

The number of deaths has increased since 1900, but we all know that the population increased, too. Thus, from the data given we should not conclude that Americans of 1970 are less healthy than Americans in 1900.

To generate comparable indices, we need to know the population for each of those years. In this example, the population that has the potential of dying in the given year is the **population at risk** or **PAR.** In general, this term identifies the population that can produce the health event under study.

However, numbers of deaths or other health events *are* of interest to those concerned with the quantity of the outcome—such as life insurance administrators, health planners, hospital administrators, and morticians. Therefore, the numbers of health events are important to those providing services specific to the health event. For example, knowing the number of diabetics or mentally retarded persons in a population can guide administrators in estimating the required amounts of service and staff for cases, the quantities of drugs required, and the size and types of physical facilities needed to care for the persons affected.

But the number of health events does not give us a basis for comparing one population with another since the two populations at risk may be very different. In order to compare the death experiences of the US population at different periods, we must allow for the difference in population size. This is why census years are chosen, for they are points at which the most accurate population counts are available.

Thus, population counts can help us correctly compare and answer the questions in Exercise 1.1.

☐ Calculate the mortality (death) rates per 1,000 population for the years given and complete Table 1.2.

Exercise 1.2

Table 1.2   **Total Population, Deaths, and Death Rates in Death Registration States, USA, for Selected Years**

Year	Persons (in millions)	Deaths (in 1,000s)	Annual death rate (per 1,000)
1900	19.9	343	
1920	86.1	1,118	
1940	131.7	1,417	
1960	179.3	1,711	
1970	203.2	1,921	

Source: *Vital Statistics of the United States, 1970.* vol. II, part A, pp 6-16. US Department of Health, Education, and Welfare, United States Public Health Service, National Center for Health Statistics, 1974.

Comment

As you read the heading to Table 1.2, you should have noted that the years chosen are the same as in Table 1.1, the numbers of population are in millions, and the numbers of deaths are in thousands.

In fact, the populations of these registration states had increased. That is why you were asked to allow for these changes in population size by calculating rates, before correctly answering Exercise 1.1.

Table 1.3 gives the correct rates for completing Table 1.2.

In order to compute these rates, first divide the number of events (deaths) by the number of persons exposed to the risk of the event (the population of those states for that given year). Then multiply that result by 1,000 in order to get death rate per 1,000 population.

The mortality rate is, in effect, a statement of the probability or likelihood of dying within a given time period. Thus, for the year 1940, out of a population of 131.7 million, 1.417 million (or 1,417 thousand) died, so the calculated probability of dying in 1940 is 1.417/ 131.7 = 0.0108.

Table 1.3   **Annual Death Rates, Death Registration States, USA, for Selected Years**

Year	Death rate (per 1,000, to nearest decimal)
1900	17.2
1920	13.0
1940	10.8
1960	9.5
1970	9.5

Source: Same as for Table 1.1.

Because these probabilities usually turn out to be small numbers, they are multiplied by some constant such as 100, 1,000, 10,000, or 100,000 to make the numbers more readable. Multiplying our probability of 0.0108 by 1,000, we get 10.8, which is the death rate per 1,000 persons for the year 1940. One interpretation is that, out of every 1,000 persons in the population, on the average 10.8 of them died during the year. These death rates for populations are called **crude death rates** since they include the entire population and are not reflective of any subpopulations, such as only females or only people aged 20 to 29.

The death rate, or any rate you calculate, is a probability statement that estimates the frequency of occurrence of a health event in a group. Although it may be used to show the likelihood that a given event will occur in the *group*, the rate will not pick out which *individuals* in the group will experience the health event.

Barring unusual circumstances such as wars or epidemics, which can cause an unusually high number of deaths, it is reasonable to apply this mortality rate to future years for purposes of prediction. This process is called **extrapolation.**

Determining the population at risk may not be as simple a matter as it appears. For example, the number of persons exposed to the risk of dying, the denominator in our equation, was the number of persons alive in the death registration states on January 1, 1940, plus all persons born in those states during 1940, with adjustments made for persons who moved in and out of or spent only part of the year in those states. A common solution to this problem of determining the population at risk is to estimate the population at the *midpoint* of the interval that the rate covers. For 1940 for example, the population at risk would be the population of those death registration states on July 1, 1940. Because the census is taken only once every 10 years, finding the population for intervening dates becomes a problem. However, there are statistical techniques for estimating the population at any given time, provided that census data from recent years are available.

Exercise 1.3

☐ Using the death rates in Table 1.3 for comparison, do you think Americans were healthier in 1970 than in 1900?
☐ What makes you think that?

Comment

Clearly the rates have declined. We can compare them because they have a common base: per 1,000 population at risk in each of the years. However, the changes in these rates *could* result from additional differences in the composition of the population being compared over time, differences other than the size of the population at risk. These differences could increase or decrease the likelihood of death in one or more of the populations and hence influence the numerators of our rates.

Let us consider, now, what other characteristics of populations could influence the number among the population at risk who experienced the event in this example. It would be logical to assume that these characteristics—such as increased age, an epidemic, a war, initiation of a new health program—would have to increase or decrease the likelihood of death, or whatever health outcome is being considered.

Exercise 1.4

Read Table 1.4.

☐ For the years shown in Tables 1.1 and 1.2 (1900, 1920, 1940, 1960, and 1970), did the US population change with respect to the distribution of age?
☐ What were the changes?

Table 1.4   **Percentage Age Distribution of the US Population, for Selected Years**

Year	Total	Under 5	5–19	20–44	45–64	65 and over
1860	100	15.4	35.8	35.7	10.4	2.7
1880	100	13.8	34.3	35.9	12.6	3.4
1900	100	12.1	32.3	37.8	13.7	4.1
1920	100	11.0	29.8	38.4	16.1	4.7
1940	100	8.0	26.4	38.9	19.8	6.9
1960	100	11.3	27.1	32.2	20.1	9.3
1970	100	9.4	28.4	31.7	20.6	9.9

Source: US Bureau of the Census: *Statistical Abstract of the United States, 1964*, ed 85. Washington, DC, 1964 and *Census, 1970*, Table 49, p I-263.

Comment

Did you read the title of Table 1.4? This one tells us that the table's contents concern the US population for certain years and its age composition. The data are presented in a percentage distribution; that is, the percentage of each year's population that is made up by each age category. Thus, 15.4% (first row and third column of Table 1.4) means that for each 100 persons living in the US in 1860, 15.4 were under five years old. Another way of saying that is, of all persons living in the US in 1860, 15.4% of them were under five years old. You should be able to make similar statements for the other percentage figures in the table.

Advice to beginners in table reading: Read and mentally "digest" the title. Then, within the table read in one direction first and then in the other direction—for example, by rows and then columns. Reading Table 1.4 across the rows, we see that in the year 1900, of each 100 persons, over one-third of them were in the 20 to 44 age group, about one-third were in the 5 to 19 age group, and 4.1% were in the 65 and over age group.

Reading down the column labeled "under 5," we see that for 1920, 1940, 1960, and 1970, the percentage of the population under five years declined and then rose, and fell again in 1970. At no time has it returned to the 1900 figure. Thus, the proportions of young children are different in our chosen years.

The other most striking differences are seen in the respective proportions of the population in the oldest age category. The percentage of the population over 64 years of age rose from 4.1% in 1900 to 9.9% in 1970. Because the total population has also increased, there have to be more older people around than in earlier decades. However, if there are also fewer younger people around, the percentages in other age categories could still increase since each row (each year) adds up to 100%.

Exercise 1.5

Read Table 1.5.

Table 1.5   **Death Rates by Age, USA, 1970**

Age (years)	Death rate (per 1,000)
Under 1	21.4
1–4	0.8
5–34	1.0
35–44	3.1
45–54	7.3
55–64	16.6
65 and over	58.9
All ages	9.5

Source: *Vital Statistics of the United States, 1970*, vol II, Mortality, part A, pp 6-17 and part B, pp 7-93, US Department of Health, Education, and Welfare, United States Public Health Service, National Center for Health Statistics, 1974.

□ What is the relationship of age to death?

Comment

Note that Table 1.5 gives death rates, by age, in the 1970 US population. When each death rate is specific to a particular age group, they are called **age-specific death rates.** The death rates you calculated in Exercise 1.2, in contrast, are rates for entire populations, called *crude death rates* because they are the simplest. Just as with crude oil, there are more varied uses for the refined product (in our case, specific death rates). The crude death rate makes no allowance for any differences in the characteristics or in the composition of the populations at risk that are being compared.

The age-specific death rates in Table 1.5 confirm the generally known fact that death rates for various age categories are not equal to one another. Table 1.5 shows that the death rate for infants is high; the death rate decreases and remains low for ages 1 to 34; then the rates progressively increase with increasing age. Note that the death rate does not increase progressively with age immediately after birth and that each age interval in Table 1.5 does not have the same number of years. Hence, the relationship between age and the death rate is nonlinear (it is not a straight line).

Exercise 1.6

For practice, calculate the age-specific death rates for 1966 to complete Table 1.6.

Table 1.6   **Deaths and Populations at Risk, by Age, USA, 1966**

Age (years)	Persons* (in 100,000s)	Deaths* (in 100,000s)	Age-specific death rates (per 1,000)
Under 5	198	1.0	
5–19	580	0.4	
20–44	601	1.3	
45–64	396	4.6	
65 and over	185	11.4	
All ages	1,960	18.7	

*All figures rounded to nearest decimal.

Source: *Vital Statistics of the United States, 1966*, vol. II, Mortality, part A, pp 1-100, Department of Health, Education, and Welfare, United States Public Health Service, National Center for Health Statistics, 1968.

☐ Do these rates show a pattern of the relationship of age to death similar to the pattern we saw in Table 1.5?

Comment

Table 1.7 presents the correct age-specific death rates to complete Table 1.6. In general, the patterns are similar to those seen in Table 1.5, but there are some important observations to be made from these two tables. Note that the age categories in the two tables are different, and this itself can produce some difference in the relationship between age and death rates. For example, the youngest age category in Table 1.6 shows a death rate of 5.1 per 1,000. By broadening the youngest age category to all those under 5 years, we have combined two populations—those under 1 year of age and those 1 to 4 years of age. These two population groups have distinctly different death rates, as illustrated in Table 1.5.

In addition, note that 1966 is not a population and housing

census year. How, then, were the population figures in Table 1.6 obtained? The Census Bureau published them in one of their many publications dealing with estimation of the overall population and various subpopulations (for example, age groups) in off-census years. Their estimation techniques use information from past decennial censuses as well as results of population counts done only in a few sections of the country during off-census years.

Table 1.7   **Age-Specific Death Rates, USA, 1966**

Age (years)	Age-specific death rates (per 1,000)*
Under 5	5.1
5–19	0.7
20–44	2.2
45–64	11.6
65 and over	61.6
All ages	9.5

*All figures rounded to nearest decimal.

Exercise 1.7

In comparing the crude death rates over time in Table 1.2, we found that the rates had declined. In Table 1.4, we learned that the age distribution of the US population had changed (in fact it had aged) over the same period of time. Next we confirmed in Tables 1.5 and 1.6 that age is related to death.

- □ What is the implication of these findings for (a) the comparison of death experience over time in one population and (b) the comparison of death rates between any two or more groups?

Comment

Because our population did differ in age distribution over time, especially in the proportion of the population that was older (over 64 years of age), and because age is related to death, with old people having the highest death rate, we cannot correctly compare the crude death rates until we have done something to make the population at risk comparable on age at those different points in time.

This manipulation is necessary because a population with a larger percentage of old people almost certainly will have a larger number of deaths than a population with a smaller percentage of old people, even though the total size of these two populations is the same. Obviously the crude death rate will be higher for the population with the larger percentage of older people.

In epidemiology, we seek to determine the cause of various health outcomes. Because we know that (a) older people are more likely to die, (b) advanced age may make people more susceptible to disease if they are exposed to disease agents, and (c) older people have had more years in which to come into contact with all sorts of things, including disease agents, we reason that group differences in age may confuse or confound our comparisons of two or more populations. Such confusing characteristics or variables are called **confounding variables.**

Similarly, the crude death rate could be high in a country having few older people but a very high proportion of infants, who also have a relatively high age-specific death rate. This would describe the current situation in many less industrialized societies.

In order to make two populations comparable on age, we do not do a biological manipulation of the ages but rather a statistical manipulation by various analytical methods that are used to compare rates. In order to avoid having group differences in age confound our comparison of death rates, we must either control for age or adjust for age. In so doing, we are adjusting or controlling for compositional differences in the populations, in this example, for age. Once we have made the populations statistically similar in age, any differences we then observe with respect to death rates could not be due to age.

Exercise 1.8

☐ What is the principle illustrated by this example in regard to comparing rates among two or more populations or groups that are different in certain respects?

Comment

The overall principle is: If any two or more populations that are being compared differ on any characteristic that *is related* to the disease or health status being considered (in this instance death) and to the exposure (or potential risk factor or cause), then these differences must be taken into account in making the comparisons.

If the populations being compared differ on any characteristic that *is not related* directly or indirectly to the disease or health status being considered, one can generally disregard the differences in this characteristic when making the disease comparisons. In this event, the comparison being made would not be confounded by irrelevant characteristics. This suggests that in studying a disease or health event, we should know what characteristics, in addition to those being studied, are related to the event. A factor is potentially confounding if it is known to be associated with the outcome variable (effect) and the characteristic of the populations you are studying.

For example, if you are studying the association between obesity (exposure, cause, risk) and heart disease (effect), a potential confounding factor would be the eating of saturated fats since it is likely that obese people eat more saturated fats *and* eating saturated fats is associated with heart disease. You need to investigate this potential confounding effect in your own study by using your own data. If these known associations, for whatever reasons, are not found in your study, they can be disregarded for they do not confound your study. If, for example, your own data do not show an association of age with death (or other health outcomes), you should disregard it in your analyses. Then the question is why is age *not* a confounding variable in your study? The answer may be one or several reasons, for example, the manner of sample selection.

This knowledge about confounding variables will allow for more precision in associating disease (effects) with specific characteristics, unconfounded by other characteristics that are associated with disease but are not of interest in your study. Using available information, you can identify from other studies those factors which have been known to be associated with the health effect you are studying; these are potential confounders.

The term **effect modifier** refers to a variable that modifies the effect (disease, outcome) and is often part of the causative network, in an interactive sense. For example, if you find that the risk of a disease is twice as great in obese persons compared with lean persons, then obesity is associated with the disease. But if you then find that this risk is four times greater in obese *men* than lean *men*, as compared with twice as great in obese women than lean women, the variable sex appears to be modifying the effect measure—that is, the association of obesity and disease is different in the two sexes.

Exercise 1.9

As with age, there are other characteristics or variables in nature or the universe that generally modify many health events, including death. In studying most diseases or health events, these characteristics need to be considered when comparing groups that differ in them.

☐ What are some of these effect modifiers (characteristics or variables)?
☐ Why did you include these?

Comment

Some characteristics or variables are related to most health happenings and perhaps could be considered as "universals" or effect modifiers. Age, sex, ethnic group, social class status, and possibly mar-

ital status and occupation are examples. That is why these characteristics—especially age, ethnic origin, and sex—usually are taken
into account in making epidemiological comparisons. For example,
if there are generally differences in the occurrence of the disease between the sexes and our two comparison groups differ in their proportions of males and females, then the sex differences may confuse
our attempts to show a relationship of another characteristic with the
health event.

There are other characteristics of populations *specifically*
related to some diseases, causes of death, or health events but not to
others. Similarly, these characteristics must be considered in comparing population rates for only those specific diseases, causes of death,
or health events. Perhaps these could be called "disease- or health
event-specific" control or potentially confounding characteristics (or
variables). However, remember that, in order for these group composition characteristics to be relevant to our epidemiological considerations, they must be indirectly or directly related to the disease or health
event being studied.

If we wished, for example, to find out whether height is
related to lung cancer, we would have to consider whether short and
tall people smoked similar amounts of cigarettes or had similar occupational exposures to cancer-producing agents. Obviously, we would
do that because smoking and certain exposures are known to be related
to lung cancer. Age, sex, and perhaps other universal confounding variables would also have to be considered.

In this example, if we did not consider the cigarette smoking
patterns in the two height groups, we might establish a relationship
between height and lung cancer that might *not* be due to height but to
the difference in the amount the tall and short people smoked.

In contrast, if we wished to examine the relationship of
height to leukemia, we would not need to be concerned about cigarette
smoking patterns because, as of today, smoking is not known to be
related to leukemia. We would have to consider, however, the extent of
exposure to radiation in the short and tall people because of the known
relationship between radiation and leukemia.

Exercise 1.10

Table 1.8 gives data that will permit you to compare the death
rates for the US White population for 1951 and 1970 while controlling
on two characteristics, namely, age and sex.

Table 1.8   ***Deaths and Population for Whites, by Sex,
for Selected Age Categories, USA, 1951 and 1970***

Age (years)	Sex	1951 Population (in 1,000s)	1951 Deaths (in 1,000s)	Sex	1970 Population (in 1,000s)	1970 Deaths (in 1,000s)
Under 1	M	1,500	48.5	M	1,800	31.7
	F	1,400	35.2	F	1,700	23.2
25–29	M	5,300	9.1	M	6,600	9.9
	F	5,600	5.2	F	6,900	4.4
65–69	M	2,300	93.3	M	3,100	113.6
	F	2,400	60.4	F	3,900	67.2

Sources: US Bureau of the Census: *Statistical Abstract of the United States, 1964.* ed 85. Washington, DC, 1964. *Vital Statistics of the United States, 1970.* vol. II, Mortality, part A, pp 6-17, part B, pp 7-150. US Department of Health, Education, and Welfare, United States Public Health Service, National Center for Health Statistics, 1974.

☐ Calculate the age/sex-specific death rates per 100,000 White US population for 1951 and 1970 and present them in a table in the space below.

☐ Read your table and comment upon the relationship between sex and death.

□ Earlier in this exercise, you were asked to compare deaths among Americans over time. Using the rates presented in your table, compare the death experience of White Americans in 1951 and 1970.

Comment

Your table should resemble Table 1.9 and should have a title, the populations for each age/sex group, and the rates. It is customary to include in tables the denominators (populations) or numerators (deaths, in this table) of rates so that readers may know the size of the populations on which the rates are based. In dealing with national statistics, where the populations are known to be very large, the population figures are sometimes omitted from the table.

Recall the procedure in calculating rates of a specific nature. In this table, the rate of 3,233 per 100,000 is the age/sex-specific death rate for American White males under 1 year of age for the year 1951. It was derived by dividing the number of White males under 1 year of age who died during 1951 by the total number of White males at risk of dying (the population of White males under 1 year old living in 1951) and then multiplying that result by 100,000. That is, $3,233 = (48.5/1,500) \times 100,000$.

Table 1.9   *Death Rates per 100,000 Population for Whites,
by Sex, for Selected Age Categories, USA,
1951 and 1970*

Age (years)	Sex	1951 Population (in 1,000s)*	1951 Death rate*	Sex	1970 Population (in 1,000s)*	1970 Death rate*
Under 1	M	1,500	3,233	M	1,800	1,761
	F	1,400	2,514	F	1,700	1,365
25–29	M	5,300	171	M	6,600	150
	F	5,600	93	F	6,900	64
65–69	M	2,300	4,057	M	3,100	3,665
	F	2,400	2,517	F	3,900	1,723

Figures are rounded.

This makes the number obtained, 3,233, a specific rate for a specific age/sex/year category. It is also specific for ethnic group, because it excludes all non-Whites. Exclusion is another way of controlling characteristics in making comparisons. Note, therefore, that any interpretation you make from your table is only for Whites of selected ages.

Looking down the columns and considering each sex separately (controlling for sex), we see that, in both years, age is nonlinearly related to death for each sex. That is, the death rate decreases from the under 1 to the 25 to 29 group and then increases to the 65 to 69 group.

Looking down the columns and considering each age separately (controlling for age), we see that in both years at all ages males have a higher death rate than females. (The reason for this has not been scientifically proven as yet.)

Looking across the rows (controlling for age and sex) while comparing 1951 and 1970, we see that death rates have declined for all the age/sex groups shown in the table.

On the basis of the data in Table 1.9, controlling for age and sex, the 1970 US White population is "healthier" than the 1951 US White population in terms of having lower death rates.

Note that the use of control tables, such as Table 1.9, is only one method of controlling for the differences in characteristics between groups being compared. These specific rates (such as age- or sex-specific rates) compare groups who are similar by excluding everyone but a selected group (an age or sex group, for example). In this way, differences that you observe cannot be explained on the basis of the "specific characteristic" since the groups are similar regarding this factor. However, as we saw with Table 1.9, comparing specific rates for only two variables (age and sex) is challenging to the attention and to the eyes—just imagine the cross-eyed nightmare of making comparisons in a table with four or more variable-specific rates that have to be examined.

We can avoid that by some obvious ways—one way is to use a standard population and see what would happen in it if population A's death rates apply. Then, repeat this process using the same standard population by applying population B's rates. The calculated expected rates would be comparable and not influenced by age differences between A and B because we would be using the same standard population. Further, this would give us one adjusted rate to compare for each population instead of a number of specific rates.

Exercise 1.11

Table 1.10 shows the population and deaths in communities A and B. Calculate the age-specific and crude death rates for A and B and complete Table 1.10.

Table 1.10   **Population and Number of Deaths, by Age, Communities A and B**

Age (years)	Community A			Community B		
	Population	Deaths	Death rate (per 1,000)	Population	Deaths	Death rate (per 1,000)
Under 1	1,000	15		5,000	100	
1–14	3,000	3		20,000	10	
15–34	6,000	6		35,000	35	
35–54	13,000	52		17,000	85	
55–64	7,000	105		8,000	160	
Over 64	20,000	1,600		15,000	1,350	
Total	50,000	1,781		100,000	1,740	

☐ Compare the crude death rates of A and B.

□ Compare the age-specific death rates of communities A and B. Why are these comparisons different from the crude rates?

Comment

Your table should resemble Table 1.11. The crude rate in community A is about twice as high as in B. The age-specific rates, however, are not very different; in the older age groups and in the under 1 year group, B's rates are higher than A's.

It is apparent that this disparity between the comparison of the crude rates and the age-specific rates is due to the larger percentage of older people (over 64 years) in A; 40% of population A but only 15% of population B is 65 or older.

Table 1.11 **Population, Deaths, and Death Rate by Community and by Age**

| Age (years) | Community A | | | Community B | | |
	Population	Deaths	Death rate (per 1,000)	Population	Deaths	Death rate (per 1,000)
Under 1	1,000	15	15.0	5,000	100	20.0
1–14	3,000	3	1.0	20,000	10	0.5
15–34	6,000	6	1.0	35,000	35	1.0
35–54	13,000	52	4.0	17,000	85	5.0
55–64	7,000	105	15.0	8,000	160	20.0
Over 64	20,000	1,600	80.0	15,000	1,350	90.0
All ages	50,000	1,781	35.6	100,000	1,740	17.4

Exercise 1.12

Let us see if we can avoid the problem of differences in ages of populations, as we conjectured earlier, by using some standard. If we use a standard population (the age distribution is standard), we can apply A's age-specific rates and find out how many deaths we would expect in A and then repeat the process for population B. We can use any population we choose to be a standard. Why not use the combined population of A and B?

Table 1.12 **Standard Population by Age and Age-Specific Death Rates for Communities A and B**

Age (years)	Standard population (A and B)	Death rate in A (per 1,000)	Expected deaths at A's rates	Death rate in B (per 1,000)	Expected deaths at B's rates
Under 1	6,000				
1–14	23,000				
15–34	41,000				
35–54	30,000				
55–64	15,000				
Over 64	35,000	_____	_____	_____	_____
Total	150,000				
Age-adjusted death rate (per 1,000)					

Complete Table 1.12 by writing in the age-specific rates for community A in column 3, and for community B in column 5 (from your Table 1.10) Calculate, for each age, the number of deaths expected in the standard population if A's age-specific death rates apply (write numbers in column 4) and then if B's rates apply (column 6).

Divide the total expected deaths for A and for B by the population in the standard (150,000) to get the age-adjusted rate.

☐ Compare the age-adjusted death rates for A and B. How does this comparison differ from the comparison of the crude death rates for A and B?

Comment

Your completed table should be like Table 1.13.

Table 1.13   ***Standard Population by Age and Age-Specific Death Rates for Communities A and B***

Age (years)	Standard population	Death rate in A (per 1,000)	Expected deaths at A's rates	Death rate in B (per 1,000)	Expected deaths at B's rates
Under 1	6,000	15.0	90	20.0	120
1–14	23,000	1.0	23	0.5	11.5
15–34	41,000	1.0	41	1.0	41
35–54	30,000	4.0	120	5.0	150
55–64	15,000	15.0	225	20.0	300
Over 64	35,000	80.0	2,800	90.0	3,150
Total	150,000	35.6	3,299	17.4	3,772.5
Age-adjusted death rate (per 1,000)		22		25	

In case it is not clear, let us go through it together. There are 6,000 persons under 1 year of age in the standard population. At A's age-specific death rate (15 per 1,000), we would expect 90 deaths in this age group. At *B*'s death rate, in that age group we would expect 120 deaths. Adding all of the expected deaths at *A*'s rates yields 3,299 deaths; adding them at *B*'s rates yields 3,772.5 deaths. (The 0.5 death is a numerical reality, not 0.5 of a body!) Dividing each of the expected number of deaths by the standard population (150,000) gives an age-adjusted rate of 22 per 1,000 for *A* and 25 per 1,000 for *B*.

You may not realize it but you have just done an age adjustment of rates, using the **direct method.**

Rates are routinely adjusted for age because age is by far the most important attribute or characteristic related to death and disease. It may be necessary—and it is possible—to use the direct method to adjust for additional variables, such as race and sex. By now, you know that to do age adjustment, you need age-specific rates for the populations being studied. A standard population is always available. Here we used the combined populations as our standard population; some researchers use the US population of a given census year, such as the 1940 population. Also, there is such a thing as a world standard population. Remember, the standard population is used for comparative purposes only. It stands to reason that one cannot use two different standard populations in adjusting rates.

Now let us go on to the interpretation of the age-adjusted death rates. Recall that the crude death rates for communities *A* and *B* were 35.6 per 1,000 and 17.4 per 1,000, respectively. So it *appeared* that community *A* was in much worse shape than community *B*. However, noting that community *A* had a much larger proportion of older people than community *B*, we then calculated age-adjusted death rates for each community—22 per 1,000 for *A* and 25 per 1,000 for *B*. The age-adjusted death rates are fairly close to each other; in fact the rate is slightly higher in community *B*. The difference between the adjusted rates of 22 and 25 *cannot* be due to age differences in the two populations since we have adjusted (or controlled statistically) for age. The difference may reflect an actual difference in death rates in the two populations, *or* it may be due to some other confounding factor or variable for which we have not adjusted (such as sex or race).

Exercise 1.13

The other method of adjustment that we will consider is the reverse of the direct method. Instead of using a standard population and specific rates from the comparison populations, we use standard rates and apply them to our comparison populations. This is called the **indirect method** of rate adjustment.

□ a. From Table 1.14, calculate the expected number of deaths in community A if the standard rates apply (here we are using B's rates as standard) and complete Table 1.14.

Table 1.14   **Population and Expected Deaths of Community A by Age, and Standard Death Rates by Age**

Age (years)	Population in A	Standard death rate (per 1,000)	Expected deaths in A at standard rates
Under 1	1,000	20.0	
1–14	3,000	0.5	
15–34	6,000	1.0	
34–54	13,000	5.0	
55–64	7,000	20.0	
Over 64	20,000	90.0	
Total	50,000	17.4	

□ b. There were 1,781 deaths *observed* (called O) in Community A (see Table 1.10). How many deaths were *expected* (called E) in community A by applying the standard death rates?

□ c. Compare the number of deaths observed (O) in community A with the number expected (E) by calculating what is called the **Standardized Mortality Ratio (SMR),** the ratio of observed deaths in community A to expected deaths in A (O/E).

Comment

a. Your calculations should be as shown in Table 1.15.

Table 1.15   ***Population and Expected Deaths of Community A by Age, and Standard Death Rates by Age***

Age (years)	Population in A	Expected deaths in A at standard rates
Under 1	1,000	20.0
1–14	3,000	1.5
15–34	6,000	6.0
35–54	13,000	65.0
55–64	7,000	140.0
Over 64	20,000	1,800.0
Total	50,000	2,032.5

Just for review, the number *20* expected deaths is obtained by 1,000 x 20/1,000 and the number *1.5* expected deaths is obtained by 3,000 x 0.5/1,000.

b. The expected (E) number of deaths in community A at standard rates is 2,032.5.

c. The SMR for community A is 1,781/2,032.5 = 0.876, or 88%. Thus, A has fewer deaths than expected, if we assume that community B's age-specific death rates are operating in community A.

In order to compare two populations using the indirect method, calculate an SMR for each population and then compare the two. The SMR for community A is 0.876. The SMR for community B will turn out to be 1.00, since the standard rates are the age-specific death rates of community B. So in comparing 0.876 to 1.00, the death rate (adjusted for age) is slightly lower in community A.

Exercise 1.14

☐ In summary, jot down the basic need for age adjustment when comparing death rates in various populations.

☐ Also, jot down the basic steps in age adjustment (or sex or race or whatever) via the direct method and the indirect method.

Comment

It is important that you understand age adjustment, which is a basic statistical technique often used in epidemiology.

1. Age-adjusted rates, using either method, permit a comparison of rates while controlling any confounding due to age. Of course if you wish to see the association of age with death or the effect you are studying, compare the age-specific rates.

2. **Adjusted rates** are not real rates that describe an actual occurrence, but rather rates that would occur under certain assumptions.

3. Age adjustment provides one rate per population to compare and is preferable to several age-specific comparisons.

4. The direct method of age adjustment uses a standard population and applies the age-specific rates of the populations being compared to determine the expected number of events (deaths) in the standard population. This method requires that the age-specific rates be available for each of the populations to be compared and that they be based on numbers that are not too small (a guideline is at least five deaths or events per age category).

5. The indirect method of age adjustment is used if the number of observed deaths or events per age category is small or if age-specific rates are not available. Here standard rates are applied to the populations being compared in order to calculate the expected number of deaths, which is to be compared with the observed number of deaths. The ratio of observed number of events to expected number of events is called, as you can understand, a *standardized* (you have used standard rates) *mortality* (or morbidity if sickness and not death is being studied) *ratio*, or *SMR* for short.

Summary

The methods that were covered in Chapter 1 are fundamental to epidemiology. Make sure you understand the following points before proceeding to the next chapter.

1. The development of death registration states as they affect the interpretation of death rates over time.

2. The possible value to health services administrators of knowledge about the number of health events in their populations, as well as the limitations in using these numbers in epidemiology.

3. Calculation and interpretation of crude rates, and their limitations.

4. Calculation and interpretation of characteristic-specific rates (such as age/sex-specific death rates) and their relevance in comparing health experiences of groups.

5. Reading tables.

6. Construction of tables and presentation of data in tabular form.

7. Controlling for the effects of confounding characteristics (such as age) in making group comparisons either through control tables or adjustment.

What you have learned in this exercise is basic. Once you have managed it, we hope with some enjoyment, then you are well on your way.

References and Further Reading Sources

This itemized list refers you to readings that will further your learning. The numbers listed correspond to the main reference list at the end of this manual.

Topic	Reference number	Pages
Nature of epidemiology	13	81–82
	27	1–7
	30	369–383
	38	1–16
Sources of health data	13	55–66
	31	32–36
	38	73–102
	40	160–183
Age adjustment of rates	16	47–51
	27	181–184
	29	201–219
	36	75–83
	40	146–153
Rates and ratios	27	8–15
	38	57–72
	45	265–269
Effect modifiers and confounding variables	27	177–180
	43	(article)
	50	(article)

Prevalence or Cross-Sectional Method: One Epidemiological Strategy

2

This chapter considers one method of applying epidemiological concepts and principles, with some assessment of the method's strengths and weaknesses. The **cross-sectional method** is a way of *describing the distributions (or frequency distributions) of health characteristics in populations and the associations of the health characteristics with other variables.* It will tell us what sorts of groups have more or less of certain disorders, indices of health, or behaviors of interest.

Emphasis is placed on the sorts of conclusions that can or cannot be derived from data obtained by this strategy. This method will not tell us *why* these health differentials exist. Therefore, it is not used to test hypotheses about causation of disease. However, it can be used to generate hypotheses. It can also be used to describe situations, assist planners and administrators of services, and initiate programs and their evaluation.

Correct interpretation of tabulated data is emphasized again since this is a sine qua non of epidemiological expertise.

Exercise 2.1

"Doctor," explained the parent, "Johnny has a headache and joint pains."

"Yes," replied Dr. Smart. "This condition is commonly found here in the town."

□ How would Dr. Smart gain that impression, and is it necessarily scientifically correct?

Write down your answer in the space on the next page, then read the following discussion.

Comment

Dr. Smart probably expressed a subjective impression or hunch from her clinical practice. She may have developed it as a result of seeing a number of similar cases or based on the hearsay of colleagues. She may be correct; such hunches often have determined important health action and research activity. It is possible, however, that Dr. Smart has a reputation for her skill in dealing with such cases, and therefore sees more of these cases than other doctors in the town. For these and other reasons, Dr. Smart may be expressing a biased opinion.

Clearly it is important, prior to any health action, to confirm such a statement accurately and scientifically, to find out whether "the condition" really is common in that community. For comprehensive health programs to be scientifically planned, the relative frequencies of other health states that may be common in that town or community are also of interest.

Exercise 2.2

☐ How would one attempt scientifically or objectively to confirm Dr. Smart's opinion that the condition was common in the town?

Comment

It would seem obvious that this could be achieved by obtaining data from facilities that treat sick people. But many sick people diagnose and treat themselves and never appear at health facilities; others go to physicians who in turn may not write down the diagnosis or may write it illegibly; still other people are treated by nurses, pharmacists, dentists, chiropractors, ministers of religion, parents, grandparents, or herbalists, who are not affiliated with a health facility. So data obtained from facilities or providers of medical services may yield very incorrect or less than complete information about the community.

Another possibility is to examine everyone in the population of interest to discover if they suffer from this "common" disorder. In this example, the population is the town where Dr. Smart resides. If the population is large, it is not feasible in terms of time and money to examine every person in the population. So in many cases, a sample is selected from the population, and only the persons in the sample are examined. The sample is selected in such a manner that it is representative of the population, even though it is usually much smaller than the population.

Clearly presence of the disorder must be discernible by ethically possible, scientific methods if the frequency of the disorder is to be systematically documented. However, some chronic diseases have clinical remissions, periods of freedom from any signs or symptoms. During such periods, these persons ("cases") may be called "noncases." Studies of conditions with remissions, such as rheumatoid arthritis, peptic ulcer, and asthma, will require special attention.

We should first define the condition under study. In this example, it would be the illness that Johnny has, but it could be a health behavior (such as immunization) or health-related behavior (such as number of cigarettes smoked). The definition must be practical, feasible, measurable, ethically derived, and the best available. Reading published material often aids in this aspect. Second, we would count the number of persons among the population or among the sample selected who showed the diagnostic criteria defined for this condition.

Sampling note: We repeat; in epidemiology, as in all other population-based sciences, we can study a total population or a sample of it. A science unto itself, sampling relies on a variety of methods. It is important to realize that the inferences and generalizations that are possible from any sample are directly related to the method of selecting the sample. The references to sampling given at the end of this exercise will be understandable and useable by a nonmathematically oriented user of this manual. If in doubt about sampling techniques and their utility, ask someone who knows more than you do.

Exercise 2.3

□ To what use can we put our knowledge of the number of persons in a community affected by a health problem, that is, the number of cases?

Comment

With respect to chronic disease, knowing the number of cases would tell us the load of illness carried in this community; it would indicate how many hospital beds, clinics, nurses, drugs, and so on, the area needed. This type of information is of great utility to health planners and administrators. The information reflects merely the frequency of various illnesses, regardless of the size of population; it indicates how many cases are in need of services.

Clinical impressions, such as Dr. Smart's, may extend to hunches about which group or aggregate of persons has more or less of the disease. Confirmation of such differences existing in subpopulations would lead, among other things, to speculation as to why such differences exist. In this exercise, we are concerned with a method of scientific observation that documents the presence or absence of a health attribute in persons who concurrently have one or more other characteristics. While the load of cases is important, however, we know that we cannot directly compare the numbers of cases in different groups because the groups may differ in size of population or in other relevant attributes. We learned about that idea in Chapter 1.

Exercise 2.4

☐ a. What measures do we need in order to establish the extent of a prevailing health state or disease and to be able to compare the states of health of different groups at a point in time?

☐ b. Logically, what would you call those measures?

☐ c. What would be the numerator and the denominator for such a rate of "olivitis" (a fictitious disease) in women aged 36 years on October 29, 1979?

Comment

a. As we learned in Chapter 1, in order to account for the different size of groups at risk and make further comparisons possible, we need rates. Hence, we need to know the number of persons who have the health state or disease, and we need to know the size of the group, that is, the size of the PAR.

b. In this instance, we could logically call the rates *point* (at a point in time when assessment is made) *prevalence* (from the word "prevailing," to be current, to exist) *rates* (you do know why they are rates). Because we have reduced the number of cases to rates, we can compare these in order to see if one group with certain characteristics has more or less of the health condition than another group without those characteristics.

Point prevalence rates are obtained by conducting a prevalence or cross-sectional survey. The survey merely describes the existence of the condition studied, the extent to which it prevails in various groups at the time of assessment. It is, in fact, a point-in-time prevalence, much like an Instamatic snapshot of a community's health state, as contrasted with a movie film, which takes a picture over time.

c. The numerator is the number of 36-year-old females on October 29, 1979 who suffer from olivitis. The denominator is the PAR, all females aged 36 on October 29, 1979. Recall that the PAR could be the entire population or a sample from that population, depending upon what you examined.

Once again, as in Chapter 1, we would multiply by some constant, often 1,000.

Exercise 2.5

☐ What does the establishment of these prevalence rates tell us, in terms of (a) health care programs, (b) other aspects of scientific health practice, and (c) further epidemiological pursuits?

Comment

a. The prevalence rates indicate among which groups to look for cases if you need to find cases for care, which groups need what sort of medical care, nursing care, and so on, and the differential need among groups for staff and budget. Thus, the point prevalence rate will indicate priority groups for health and medical care, including case finding.

b. Further, if a project aims to reduce the load of illness in a community, point prevalence rates (PPR) will serve as baseline indices for subsequent evaluation of health and medical care services in the groups served.

c. As indicated in Chapter 1, a rate is a probability statement. A prevalence rate gives the likelihood of cases existing in certain groups. In subsequent epidemiological pursuits, it would tell us how many people we would have to examine on the average to find a desired number of cases for study. Thus, if we wished to carry out a study on 100 cases of olivitis, and we know the PPR was 2%, then we would need to examine at least 5,000 people in order to be reasonably sure of obtaining 100 cases of olivitis.

The field of sampling, as mentioned earlier, has techniques to determine the exact sample size required so that the probability is 0.90 or 0.95 or whatever that at least 100 cases would be found, for any given PPR. These sampling considerations are often neglected in planning surveys or studies.

Exercise 2.6

You established that

Point prevalence rate =

$$\frac{\text{Number of cases of disease}}{\text{Number in population at risk}} \times \text{Constant}$$

where the number in PAR are those persons eligible to be in the numerator.

☐ What factors, therefore, could influence point prevalence rates and make them higher or lower? (This needs simple logical thinking.)

Comment

The numerator (number of cases) can be increased by an increase in the occurrence of new cases (incidence) or by keeping cases alive longer through improved care. Curing them, however, will make them noncases. Similarly, a rise in deaths from this disease will reduce the number of cases prevailing or found living and this, as with cure, will reduce the PPR. Further, if cases migrate—"take their sinuses to Phoenix or their heart disease to Houston"—then selective migration will cause fewer cases to be found in some places and more cases to be found in Phoenix and Houston. Thus, out-migration of cases decreases the PPR and, similarly, in-migration of cases increases the numerator and thus increases the point prevalence rate.

The denominator can also be affected. Because healthy immigrants inflate the denominator and not the numerator, they will decrease the PPR. As shown in Figure 2.1, the point prevalence rate can be seen as see-saw, a scale, or any other kind of balance you can dream up.

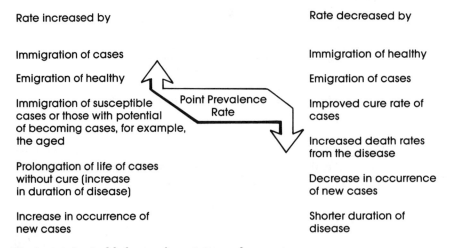

Rate increased by

Immigration of cases

Emigration of healthy

Immigration of susceptible cases or those with potential of becoming cases, for example, the aged

Prolongation of life of cases without cure (increase in duration of disease)

Increase in occurrence of new cases

Point Prevalence Rate

Rate decreased by

Immigration of healthy

Emigration of cases

Improved cure rate of cases

Increased death rates from the disease

Decrease in occurrence of new cases

Shorter duration of disease

Figure 2.1 Logical balance of a point prevalence rate.

Exercise 2.7

☐ Why is this rate called "point prevalence"?

Comment

In point prevalence studies (also called *cross-sectional stud-ies*), each subject is assessed only once at one point in time. Theoret-ically, such a cross-sectional survey could be completed within a short period of time if we had many observers. In reality, such studies may take months or even years to complete. But each person is assessed only once, and at that point, the existence of the disease and other characteristics are rated in that person.

You will come across the term **period prevalence.** This is the number (or rate) of cases found over a specified period of time, say one year. Cases are counted for period prevalence even if they die, migrate, recur as episodes, and so on, during the period. Thus, if a case is found in the population in January and dies or departs or is cured by March, it is counted in the year's period prevalence, but that case would not be included in a point prevalence in June of that year. Similarly, period prevalence includes cases current during the specified period regard-less of when they became a case or ceased to be a case.

Thus, period prevalence will equal a point prevalence at the start of the time period and all new cases (incidence) during the period, divided by the average population during the period. Period preva-lence, then, gives a picture of the load of illness in a group over a period of time. However, it is of very limited usefulness in epidemiology and will not be emphasized in this manual. General use of the term "prev-alence" suggests point prevalence, unless otherwise indicated. A num-ber of good references on prevalence study strategy are listed at the end of Chapter 2.

Exercise 2.8

In 1960 a community survey in Evans County, Georgia, produced the following findings from examinations of the population 40 to 74 years old. The entire population was measured rather than a sample from the population.

Table 2.1 Cases of CHD,* Population 40 to 74 Years Old, Evans County, Georgia, 1960

Number examined	Cases of CHD	Persons free from CHD
2,216	130	2,086

*CHD = coronary heart disease. Cases include "definite," "probable," and "possible" cases of CHD.

Source: McDonough JR, Hames CG, Stulb SC, and Garrison GE: Coronary heart disease among Negroes and Whites in Evans County, Georgia. *J. Chronic Dis,* 18:443, 468, 1965. Copyright 1965, Pergamon Press, Ltd.

□ a. From Table 2.1, calculate the point prevalence rate of CHD among persons 40 to 74 years old in Evans County in 1960.

□ b. To what use can those concerned with health care put this information?

Comment

a. Point prevalence rate is the number of cases found, divided by the PAR, that is, those eligible to be a case.

$$\text{PPR} = \frac{130}{2216} \times 1,000 = 58.6 \text{ per } 1,000$$

b. It tells us that in 1960 almost 6% (5.86 per 100) of the Evans County population 40 to 74 years old had coronary heart disease. For this county, and for communities similar to it, this estimate tells us the load of CHD. This may permit, in turn, estimating needed facilities and funds, the extent of employment disability, as well as other ramifications of this disease. It also could indicate whether CHD is more prevalent in Evans County than other disorders and thereby contributes information to help set priorities for decisions regarding health services.

Further, it does indicate the likelihood of finding a case. Thus, we know that in Evans County, in 1960, if an epidemiological study of CHD needed 30 cases for its sample, we would have to examine about 500 persons in the age category 40 to 74 years.

Also, if a program is instituted to reduce the number of cases in the county over the next few years and if it is successful, clearly a repeat cross-sectional study years later among persons 40 to 74 years old should find CHD at a point prevalence rate of less than 6%. However, this reduction in prevalence should occur because of "good" things happening that reduce PPR (fewer new cases) and not "bad" things (increased death rates), as per our logical balance.

Exercise 2.9

The same study in Evans County found the following age distribution of the cases of CHD among White males aged 40 to 74 years.

☐ From Table 2.2, can you calculate the point prevalence rate of CHD in White males of Evans County? If so, what is the rate per 1,000? If not, why not?

Table 2.2   *Age Distribution of Cases of CHD,* White*
Males, 40 to 74 Years Old, Evans County, 1960

Age (years)	Cases of CHD
40–49	12
50–59	19
60–69	29
70–74	11
Total 40–74	71

*Cases include "definite," "probable," and "possible" CHD.
Source: Same as Table 2.1.

Comment

You cannot calculate the PPR because a rate needs a denominator from which the numerator arises. We have the number of cases of CHD in White males 40 to 74 years old (71), but no denominator of the total population of White males 40 to 74 years old.

Exercise 2.10

□ a. Does Table 2.2 demonstrate an association between age and CHD prevalence?

□ What makes you think that?

☐ b. What do you understand by the term *association*?

☐ c. What additional data would help you decide if there is an association of age with CHD?

Comment

a. The number of cases does increase with age up to 69 years, but so might the population in each age category. So, as it stands, no test or statement can be made of an age association with CHD prevalence until we can calculate age-specific prevalence rates. The general rules hold—comparisons of groups or categories (for example, age) demand rates, and not cases or numerator data only. And comparison is central to epidemiology.

b. An **association** between two variables implies that as one variable (characteristic) changes, there is a concomitant or resultant change in the quantity or quality of the other variable. In this instance, an associaion of age with CHD would simply mean different rates of CHD for different age groups.

c. Clearly, we need to know how many persons were examined in each age category, that is, the PAR in each age category.

Exercise 2.11

Table 2.3   **Age Distribution of White Males,
40 to 74 Years Old, Evans County, 1960**

Age (years)	Persons
40–49	254
50–59	219
60–69	139
70–74	52
Total 40–74	664

Source: Same as Table 2.1.

☐ From Tables 2.2 and 2.3, do you find that age is associated with CHD prevalence? Show the figures that make you think that.

Comment

Using Tables 2.2 (for the numerator) and 2.3 (for the denominator), you can calculate the age-specific prevalence rates shown in Table 2.4.

Table 2.4   **Age-Specific Prevalence Rates, White Males,
40 to 74 Years Old, Evans County, 1960**

Age (years)	Rate per 1,000
40–49	$(12/254) \times 1{,}000 = 47.2$
50–59	$(19/139) \times 1{,}000 = 86.7$
60–69	$(29/139) \times 1{,}000 = 208.6$
70–74	$(11/52) \times 1{,}000 = 211.5$
Total 40–74	$71/664 \times 1{,}000 = 106.9$

Source: Sames as Table 2.1.

It is obvious that the age-specific rates go up with increased age, which is a **positive association** of age with CHD prevalence rates. Note also that the rates of CHD do not increase steadily, but there is a big difference in the rates of the two older categories compared to the younger ones. As you well know by now, these rates are called age-specific point prevalence rates, for they pertain to each age category separately, or specifically.

Exercise 2.12

☐ What are the implications of the association of CHD with a characteristic such as age in comparing CHD rates found between two or more groups?

Comment

From Chapter 1, you learned that because age is associated with CHD prevalence, age modifies CHD prevalence and is therefore a potential confounder in all prevalence studies of CHD. Confirmation of the confounding effect arises from each study's data. Then, if confirmed, all subsequent analyses on CHD must control or adjust for age differences in groups being compared. In doing so, one avoids making erroneous interpretations of differences between two groups that, in fact, may be due only to the differences in their age composition.

Thus, for example, if we want to see whether obese men have higher CHD rates than nonobese men, we must ensure comparability of age in the two weight groups before we are able to test or establish an association of obesity with CHD. It is likely that our study will confirm that age is associated with obesity and with CHD.

Exercise 2.13

☐ What sorts of hypotheses, considerations, or processes could explain an association of age with disease prevalence?

Comment

If the association is positive (as age increases, point prevalence increases), then the following explanations are some of the possibilities.

First, it may have something to do with biological aging—with the body changes inexorably produced by age that make people rush for hair transplants, face lifts, creams, and other supports.

Second, the older one gets, the longer one is exposed to all sorts of stresses—pollution, beer, parents-in-law, taxes—and this accumulation of exposure may produce higher rates in older people. That is, the more one has of a deleterious thing, the more likely the illness is to occur.

Third, the death rate of cases (referred to as the case fatality ratio) may be greater in the young than in the old. That is, the disease is more fatal or of shorter duration in the younger ages so fewer cases are found in younger persons or new cases of the disease are less common in younger ages, so young people have lower rates.

Note: The **case fatality ratio (CFR)** is the number of deaths from the specified disease in a time period divided by the PAR. In this instance, PAR is the number of *cases* of the disease during the same period. For example:

Annual case fatality ratio for CHD =

$$\frac{\text{Number of deaths from CHD in 1970}}{\text{Number of cases of CHD in 1970}} \times 1,000$$

Notice that the numerator is the same as an annual CHD death rate, but the denominator in the case fatality ratio is *cases*, not population. A CFR can be specific to age, sex, ethnic group or any other characteristic. Also, the CFR is sensitive to activities and procedures done to prevent death of cases and often reflects aspects of quality of care, be it medical, nursing, hospital coronary care units, etc. In that sense, it can be used as an evaluative index of care of cases of the programs; a lower CFR means "better" care. Note, however, that if care is better for old people—their case fatality ratio drops, and they stay alive longer, without being cured or killed—then more of them will exist for a prevalence study, and the prevalence rate will be larger than it would be if the CFR remained high.

Fourth, it may be that the particular group of older people with the higher prevalence rate at the time of the prevalence study always had the high rate, compared to other ages, even when they were of a younger age. This is suggestive of a special age group going through life with a high rate of an illness and carrying this characteristic with them into successive age categories over time—a phenomenon called a **cohort effect.** If this were the case, the high rate, for example, would be among 40-year-olds in 1950, among 50-year-olds in 1960, among 60-year-olds in 1970, and so forth.

Fifth, it is possible that there is, in reality, no increase of disease with age but that the age association is due to early death from other causes of the healthier persons. This, in effect, leaves the unfit to live long enough to have the CHD in older ages. This phenomenon usually is called **selective survival/mortality.**

Rates of most but not all medical disorders go up with age. If the association of age with the disorder is negative, if the prevalence rate declines with advancing age, the previous logical possibilities still apply but with the appropriate modifications.

As an aside, by now if you want to add the possibility that another variable (some confounder) is producing the association of age with CHD, you may be correct. Generally, however, age is a very common confounder in studies, which is why our examples of adjustment or characteristic-specific calculations, addressed age.

Exercise 2.14

In pursuing a possible association of CHD with physical activity, the same investigators in the Evans County survey compared the prevalence rates among White male farm owners who did and did not do their own farm work and found the results listed in Table 2.5.

Table 2.5   **Prevalence of CHD Among White Male Farm Owners, 40 to 74 Years Old, by Physical Activity of Work, Evans County, 1960**

Category of activity	Persons examined	Cases of CHD	Prevalence rate (per 1,000)	Age-adjusted prevalence rates (per 1,000)
Not physically active	89	14	157.3	126
Physically active	90	3	33.3	36

Source: Same as Table 2.1.

☐ a. How does the prevalence rate among White male farm owners differ between the two physical activity categories?

☐ b. Could the difference in the rates be due to age differences, with the physically active group being younger than the inactive group, and hence having a lower rate because of their younger age and not because of their activity?

☐ Why do you think that?

□ c. How do these rates compare with the prevalence rate of CHD in the total Evans County population, aged 40 to 74 (see Exercise 2.8) and the prevalence rate in all White farm owners? (This rate can be calculated from Table 2.5.)

□ d. What could explain the differences?

Comment

a. The rate is greater among the not physically active category—almost five times as great as among those in the physically active category.

b. The differences in the crude point prevalence rates could be due to age differences. However, the age-adjusted rates in Table 2.5, which control or adjust for age differences, also differ in the same direction. The adjusted rates make the two comparison groups statistically similar in age (you learned that in Chapter 1). Thus, the difference in CHD rates by activity groups is not explained by age.

c. The total population prevalence rate of CHD was 58.6 per 1,000 (see Exercise 2.8). The prevalence rate of CHD in White male farm owners, from Table 2.5, is 17/179 = 95.0 per 1,000. The rate of

White male farm owners (95.0) is higher than the prevalence rate in the total population (58.6).

     d. Because the White male farm owners had a higher prevalence rate than the total population, some other categories must have had lower rates (for example, White nonfarm owners, females, non-Whites). And/or the age distribution may be different in farm owners as compared to the total population. And/or other CHD-relevant differences may exist among farm owners compared with other groups in the population, for example that they may smoke more cigarettes than other groups.

     Time out—A moment for computational and other considerations. In calculating the prevalence rate for farm owners from Table 2.5, we hope that you did not add the two prevalence rates (157.3 and 33.3) and divide by 2. Actually, (157.3 + 33.3)/2 = 95.3, which is close to the correct answer of 95.0, is methodologically incorrect. Averaging rates assumes that each different rate contributes equally to the average; (157.3 + 33.3)/2 is an "unweighted" average, which gives an equal weight to each component of the average. You want to give an equal weight to each rate *only if* the denominators in the calculation of the different rates are all equal to each other. In Table 2.5, the denominators (or sizes of the subgroups) were 89 and 90—not too different from each other. This is why the incorrect method gave an answer of 95.3, not too far off from the correct answer of 95.0.

     Consider, however, a more extreme hypothetical possibility, where the entire population is examined.

	Persons in population	Cases	Prevalence rate (per 1,000)
Have attribute A (active)	200	100	500
Not have attribute A (inactive)	4,800	400	83.3
Totals	5,000	500	

     The prevalence rate for the entire populaton is (500/5,000) × 1,000 = 100. Averaging 500 and 83.3 yields (400 + 83.2)/2 = 291.6—quite a different result from 100. By averaging the two rates, the larger rate, 500, is given as much weight as the smaller rate, 83.3, when in fact this larger rate only applies to 200/5,000 or 4% of the entire population. To get a rate for the entire population, each rate should be weighted by the population in the subgroup associated with the given rate. For example, the rate for the overall population is

$$\frac{(200 \times 500) + (4{,}800 \times 83.3)}{200 + 4{,}800} = 500{,}000/5{,}000 = 100$$

This computational note is a reminder against human impetuousness.

You will hear or read or use the terms **dependent variable** and **independent variable.** Do not let this scientific jargon throw you; it is very simple. The dependent variable merely refers to the disease or health state that you are studying epidemiologically. In this case, it is CHD. The independent variable refers to all other characteristics of groups or environments that you are attempting to associate with the occurrence of the dependent variable. In this case, the independent variable is physical activity. These terms are used because we want to see if the occurrence of the disease or health states *depends* on other characteristics.

Exercise 2.15

Can you draw the following conclusions from Table 2.5? (Give reasons for your answers.)

☐ a. Physical work prevents CHD? Why?

☐ b. Inactivity causes CHD? Why?

☐ c. CHD causes inactivity? Why?

☐ d. Physical activity is associated with CHD? Why?

Comment

a. No, because Table 2.5 merely indicates cross-sectional rates, the coexistence at a given time of the disease and the characteristic. We neither know when the CHD commenced nor when the physical activity occurred.

b. No. For the same reason as in (a).

c. No. For the same reason as in (a).

Either (a), (b), or (c) could be factually correct, but Table 2.5 does not permit such cause-effect interpretation since it is a cross-sectional study.

d. Yes. Clearly, for as the characteristic changes, so does the rate of CHD change.

Thus, in point prevalence/cross-sectional studies, we can only make statements *of* associations. We cannot make statements *about* the associations, for example, that having a particular characteristic causes one to contract the disease. However, the associations do generate hypotheses or suggest areas for further study, both highly worthwhile outcomes of prevalence studies.

Exercise 2.16

☐ From Table 2.5, can we deduce the likelihood (risk, probability) of a "healthy" inactive White Evans County farm owner developing CHD *in the future*—after 1960, that is?

☐ What in this exercise makes you think that?

Comment

We have no idea from these data. We do not know when CHD occurred in relation to activity. It is obvious that CHD can cause inactivity as much as the reverse is possible. Scientifically, one cannot base predictions of future events (risk statements) on cross-sectional data.

Exercise 2.17

In another cross-sectional study, factors associated with acceptance of immunization against poliomyelitis were examined. Table 2.6 shows the data from a sample of community members.

Table 2.6   **Vaccine Acceptance Rates by Knowledge of the Cause of Poliomyelitis**

	Knowledge of causes of poliomyelitis		
Vaccine acceptance	"Don't know" (n = 214)	"Dirt/flies" (n = 80)	"Virus" (n = 100)
Accepted	51%	67%	78%
Did not accept	49%	33%	22%

Source: Johnson AL, et al: *Epidemiology of polio vaccine acceptance.* Monograph #3, Florida State Board of Public Health, 1962.

☐ a. How many variables are included in this table?

☐ b. What describes the numerator of the 51% in the table?

☐ c. Describe the 51% in a sentence to indicate its denotation.

☐ d. From Table 2.6 can you conclude that more accurate knowledge of the cause of polio is associated with vaccine acceptance?

☐ Why do you think that?

☐ e. Of knowledge and vaccine acceptance, which causes which?

☐ Why do you think that?

Comment

a. Two variables are included: knowledge of causes of poliomyelitis and vaccine acceptance.

b. The numerator of that 51% is the number of persons who said "Don't know" about the cause of polio *and also* accepted the vaccine.

c. Of the 214 persons who said "Don't know," 51% took the vaccine. Hence, the numerator must have been 109 persons (percentages have been rounded off).

d. Yes. The more correct the knowledge of the cause of poliomyelitis, the greater the vaccine acceptance rate. We can compare these three categories of knowledge because the data on vaccine acceptance were transformed into rates. (Percentages are rates per 100!) But do not rule out the possibility of **secondary associations** (artifactual associations produced by confounding variables, such as age, social class). Thus, if older people or upper social class people have more accurate knowlege of the cause of poliomyelitis (which is likely) *and* older people or upper social class people more often accept vaccine (which is likely), then the association of vaccine taking with knowledge may be due only to the mutual association of both knowledge and vaccine taking with age or class. This creates a secondary association between knowledge and vaccine acceptance due to the confounding variable of age or social class. That is, you may be sufficiently confused by the confounding variable age or class that you believe there is true association between knowledge and vaccine acceptance when, in fact, there may be no such association. Under such circumstances, the association between knowledge and vaccine acceptance is an artifact produced by the confounding variable.

e. We do not know from this table. Knowledge could precede and in fact motivate vaccine acceptance; the reverse could hold in that knowledge may be imparted to the vaccine takers and hence the vaccine acceptance may precede knowledge.

Exercise 2.18

In Exercise 2.17, you compared three rates of vaccine acceptance among a sample of members of a Florida community. In Exercise 2.11, you compared four rates of CHD for White males in a Georgia county. Both studies were cross-sectional surveys.

□ What potential problems are introduced when a sample from the population is used rather than the total population? Just think logically of all possibilities.

Comment

Often we use a sample in epidemiology to study health of populations because it is too time-consuming or expensive or wasteful of effort to look at the entire population. But in so doing, we still strive to get accurate estimates of the health parameters of the parent population from which the sample is taken. A **parameter** is the term used to indicate the true value of a population's health attribute, for example, a prevalence rate or an immunization acceptance rate.

Clearly, for an estimate to be accurate, the sample must be representative of the population. There are several techniques for selecting samples that approach true representation. Obviously, the larger the representative sample from the population, the more likely the estimate will be to approach the population parameter. Some researchers refer to a study of a total population as a 100% sample, which seems redundant to us.

It is unlikely that two or more samples drawn from the same population will be alike. Therefore, different samples will give different values for an estimate of the population parameter. This phenomenon is called **sampling variability.**

When one selects a sample, one attempts to have a group that is as representative as possible of the total population and large enough to reduce the sampling variability to an acceptable level. Further reference to this will be made in Chapter 12.

It is clearly important, when reading a research article, to note the size of the sample and how it was selected (is it representative?).

Exercise 2.19

☐ With an understanding now of sampling variability, what explanations could there be for the differences in polio immunization acceptance rates that we found in the sample of Floridians (Table 2.6)?

Comment

The vaccine acceptance rates in the sample could differ because (1) the population rates for these three knowledge groups are different—the population parameters differ—or (2) the samples vary, even if the population parameters for these three knowledge groups are the same. (The relevance of sampling variability to observed differences in sample rates is addressed by tests of significance, which we will discuss in Chapter 12.)

Further, differences between sample rates could arise if the samples are not representative of the populations, regardless of whether the parameters differ. Conversely, and logically, one can obtain equivalent sample rates when the parameters are not equal due to sampling variability and to nonrepresentative samples.

So there are two kinds of errors one can make by using samples. Type I error: we can find a difference in our sample rates when no difference exists among the population parameters. Type II error: we can find no difference in our sample rates when there is an actual difference between the population parameters.

Exercise 2.20

☐ Consider and list the advantages and disadvantages of the cross-sectional point prevalence study method as one of the epidemiological strategies.
☐ Advantages:

□ Disadvantages:

Comment

Advantages of Cross-Sectional/Point Prevalence Strategy

1. It is quick, requiring only a "one-time" examination/interview.

2. Thus, it is cheaper.

3. Because it indicates case loads and priorities for care, it is helpful in program planning, designing and

locating hospitals, budgeting for drugs, determining types of services, and so forth.

4. It develops associations, thereby generating hypotheses.

5. Its descriptions of the relative distributions of health and disease in populations can direct case finding priorities. Therefore, it is one of the common options used in descriptive epidemiology.

Disadvantages of Cross-Sectional/Point Prevalence Strategy

1. It does not separate cause-effect relationships in the associations established; it merely points out the relatedness of characteristics and health attributes in populations.

2. Being cross-sectional at a point in time, it deals only with survivors and those around to be found as cases.

3. When rare health conditions are being considered, this strategy is not advisable. If the prevalence rate of a disease is small, say 5 per 100,000, and one wishes to establish the association of this disease with sex, age, or any other characteristic, then one would have to examine at least 200,000 persons to find about 10 cases, which may be a lot of work for little return. For these rarer events, other strategies are available; several are dealt with in subsequent exercises in this manual.

4. It is not very useful in describing the load of cases or health events when these cases are recurrent and not countable at the "point" of the study. For studying conditions such as school or industrial absences, acute recurrent illness, and seasonal variations in illness, period prevalence studies are more appropriate.

5. Given a characteristic, it does not identify risk or future likelihood of the occurrence of the disease. Therefore, it cannot predict future health happenings.

6. It has limited utility in explosive epidemics or acute, short duration illnesses such as measles or upper respiratory infectons; a point prevalence study can miss the epidemic, which may occur and subside rapidly.

Exercise 2.21

One of the sources of error, headaches, and misunderstanding in table generation and reading is choosing the correct denominator and numerator for rates. The following data will guide you in a hypothetical experience.

This study attempts to associate weight and anxiety. A sample of persons from a population were weighed and administered a questionnaire that measures anxiety. The individuals were then categorized according to the two measures.

Table 2.7   **Persons by Weight and Anxiety Categories (Hypothetical Data)**

		Anxiety		
Weight	High	Medium	Low	Total
Overweight	125	100	25	250
Normal	75	55	20	150
Underweight	45	20	5	70
Total	245	175	50	470

Would you agree with the following statements? (If not, give your own answer.)

☐ a. The rate of high anxiety in overweight persons (125/250) is greater than the rate in underweight persons (45/245).

☐ b. The rate of medium anxiety in persons with normal weight (55/175) is less than the rate in underweight persons (20/70).

☐ c. The rate of high anxiety in the whole population is 245/470, or about 52%.

☐ d. The rate of overweight in the medium anxiety category is 100/175.

☐ e. The rate of medium anxiety in overweight persons is 100/175.

☐ f. The rate of low anxiety in underweight persons (5/70) is less than the rate in those of normal weight (20/150).

Comment

Note from the table heading, that the numbers in the table represent *persons* not *rates*.

a. No. The rate of high anxiety in overweight persons is 125/250, but the rate in underweight persons is 45/70. The denominator, 70 not 245, must be the total number of persons who were underweight.

b. No. The rate of medium anxiety in persons with normal weight is 55/150, not 55/175; the rate in underweight persons is 20/70. The denominator of 150 is the total number with normal weight.

c. Yes. The numerator is 245 because it includes everyone in the 470 who has high anxiety.

d. Yes. The numerator (100) must be "medium" and "overweight"; the denominator is all of those with medium anxiety (175).

e. No. Although 100 is the correct numerator (medium anxiety and overweight), now we are concerned with all overweight persons, which is 250, not 175.

f. Yes. That is correct.

For further practice, you should look at any similar tables of rates or numbers and make statements about some of the figures. Make sure you can correctly identify numerators and denominators. Skill in table reading is invaluable in epidemiological pursuits. Clues to the correct numerators and denominators sometimes stem from the question. This may sound like an English grammar lesson, but whatever follows "of" in "the rate of" is the numerator. Whatever follows "in" or "among" denotes the denominator. Therefore, simple consideration of the question asked will help.

Whenever you want to claim that two or more rates differ from each other, and the rates are based on data from a *sample*, you will need to do a test of significance. (Again, we will learn how to do some tests of significance later on.)

Exercise 2.22

In 1960–1962, the US National Health Examination Survey found the point prevalence rates of hypertension (raised blood pressure) given in Table 2.8. These data were obtained from a sample of the US adult population.

Table 2.8   *Prevalence Rates (%) of Definite Hypertension* for White and Black† Adults, by Age and Sex: United States 1960–1962*

Age (years)	Black men	White men	Black women	White women
18–24	1.9	1.7	3.4	0.9
25–34	12.5	3.6	8.6	2.3
35–44	26.5	11.8	25.7	6.2
45–54	30.9	16.5	41.3	15.5
55–64	44.6	20.2	37.9	30.6
65–74	52.7	25.0	64.1	46.6
75–79	59.8	30.3	69.5	44.1
Total 18–79	26.7	12.8	26.6	15.3

*Definite hypertension = 160 or more mm Hg systolic blood pressure or 95 or more mm Hg diastolic blood pressure.

†The published document lists these adults as "Negro." The designation "Black" is preferred.

Source: Derived from Table 2 in *Hypertension and Hypertensive Heart Disease In Adults: United States 1960–1962.* Washington, DC, US Department of Health, Education, and Welfare, Public Health Service, National Center for Health Statistics, series 11, no. 13, 1966.

☐ a. What associations are shown in Table 2.8?

☐ b. What are the general implications of these findings for a program directed toward case finding and treatment, program evaluations, and further analyses of data or further study of hypertension?

Comment

From the heading of the table, observe that: (1) the figures given are age/ethnic group/sex-specific prevalence *rates* of hypertension and hence one can use them in comparisons; (2) there are some age categories omitted (very old and children); (3) most totals are not included so one cannot read marginals (rates for all ages, all sexes, or all ethnic groups); and (4) the numbers (numerators or denominators) are not shown so one cannot derive any other rates.

Generally, tables include denominators so that the reader can calculate numerators by applying percentages, and hence calculate other rates, if indicated. This table was extracted from a manuscript in which the numbers are given in another table. We omitted them to keep the table simpler.

a. Reading across the rows from left to right within Table 2.8, and hence controlling for age to see ethnic/sex associations, we find the following:

Comparing Blacks and Whites Within Each Sex

1. Among men, Blacks have higher rates than Whites in all age groups.

2. Among women, Blacks have higher rates than Whites in all age groups.

Therefore, Blacks have higher prevalence rates than Whites, and these ethnic differences are *not* due to the age or sex composition of the two ethnic groups.

Comparing Sexes Within Each Ethnic Group

3. Among Whites, men have higher rates than women through age 54, after which age women have higher rates than men.

4. Among Blacks, the differences by sex are not so clear. Women have higher rates than men in all age categories *except* 25 to 44 years and 55 to 64 years.

Age Association with Hypertension Prevalence
To consider the age association, one has to read the columns (from top to bottom).

5. With two exceptions, rates go up with age up to 79 years in both sex and ethnic groups. (Note: There is one exception in Black women and one in White women; the reasons for these exceptions are debatable and *may* be due to sampling variability.)

In summary, age, ethnic group, and sex are independently associated with hypertension prevalence; that is, there is an association between age and rate of hypertension in each ethnic/sex category. Ethnicity is associated with rate of hypertension in each age/sex category;

sex is associated with rate of hypertension in each age/ethnicity category; and there are also some interactive associations. For example, age and sex among Whites are interactively associated: women have lower rates of hypertension in all age categories through age 54; after that age, women have a higher rate of hypertension than men. Since the effect of sex on the rate is not the same for every age category, age and sex have an interactive association with the rate of hypertension in Whites.

This table also tells us that almost 45% of Black men 55 to 64 years old have definite hypertension, with even higher rates (remember, they are per 100 persons) among older Black men and women. In fact, even in the 1970s hypertension was a very prevalent chronic disease among Black persons in the US.

b. Applying our previous considerations, a program directed toward hypertension case finding and treatment will have the greater return per 100 persons screened among Black persons in the US. Further, these cross-sectional findings are the baseline against which to evaluate any program aimed at reducing the amount of hypertension in the country.

Because age, ethnicity, and sex are independently associated with hypertension, these characteristics are likely to be confounding variables and must be controlled or adjusted in all analyses establishing other associations with hypertension or in comparing any populations in regard to their hypertension experience. Current country-wide and worldwide programs for the detection and treatment of hypertensives, if successful, should reduce these high prevalence rates in the US and other nations.

Prevalence studies and table reading are important aspects of the epidemiological method. Acquiring some degree of ease with them is recommended. Practice reading tables so that, however complicated they are, no data presented will throw you off stride. In fact, you will end up finding interesting associations or facts often missed by authors.

Summary

Listed below are the main methodological points that were considered in Chapter 2. This chapter is rather important, for the cross-sectional or point prevalence study method is probably the most commonly used strategy in epidemiology.

1. The point prevalence rate as a measure used in descriptive epidemiology.

2. Identification and use of the correct numerators and denominators of these rates.

3. Description of the meaning of any rate.

4. The meaning of an association between two variables.

5. The need to control or adjust for differences in the groups being compared.

6. The value of knowledge of number of cases to planning services.

7. Factors that affect point prevalence rates.

8. Differences between point and period prevalence studies and rates.

9. Contributions of point prevalence studies in descriptive epidemiology toward case finding, treatment programs, and evaluation of treatment programs.

10. Control tables in controlling other variables.

11. Interpretation of tables and possible associations.

12. Advantages and disadvantages of cross-sectional studies.

13. Table generation and reading.

14. Relevance of tests of significance.

References and Further Reading Sources

Topic	Reference number	Pages
Sampling	1	39–45
	24	154–180
	29	14–24
	32	7–26
	38	250–252
	55	(entire book)
	60	16–18
	66	69–125
Cross-sectional method (prevalence study)	1	5–12
	14	(article)
	16	278–279
	27	89–102
	31	98–123
	38	61–62
	68	50–70

The Case-Control
Study Method: Looking Back

3

The cross-sectional method you learned in Chapter 2 establishes concurrent associations between characteristics and health outcomes, such as disease or health states. In contrast, the case-control research strategy inquires about antecedent characteristics and combines this with information on current health states. (In earlier years and texts, this strategy was termed "case history" method. However, to avoid confusion with the case history interview of clinical practice, "case-control" is the current preferred term. It is also called "case-referent" or "case-compeer" method.)

The prevalence rate is used in cross-sectional studies as a measure of the magnitude of the health outcome in the population of interest. The cross-sectional study design may be said to be conducted in the present, that is, "today." It does not allow us to answer the question, "Which came first, the characteristic or the condition?" Rather than contribute to the identification of cause and effect in the interpretation of associations, it merely describes what exists at the time of the prevalence study.

In an effort to support hypotheses about supposed antecedents, we may look back in time or retrospectively and ask people who have the health outcome (or effect) at the time of the study or who develop the effect during the course of the study about their past in order to find out about supposed causes. These people are the "cases." In epidemiology, we compare groups in order to establish associations. We also select a group of individuals who do *not* have or develop the health effect, a "control" group, and ask about their history of contact with or exposure to the supposed causes. Thus, this strategy is called a **case-control method.**

Exercise 3.1

☐ Before proceeding, just to put this into a broader perspective, how would you identify or support a cause and effect relationship? (There tend to be three ways; just think logically.)

Write down your answer, then read the discussion below.

Comment

1. The most obvious and easy way seems to be to obtain historical information about presumed antecedents (exposures) from patients or persons possessing the outcome or effect. This is easy because cases are available through hospitals or clinics. Thus, if we want to see whether listening to loud music in adolescence is possibly an antecedent of hypertension in adulthood, we would find adult cases of hypertension and inquire if they listened to rock music when they were adolescents. We also obtain the same history from normotensive adults for comparison. In this method, one is looking back in time to see if the presumed antecedent occurred. For this reason, the method is also called **retrospective** (from the Latin, *retro spicere*, to look back). Because we are comparing cases and controls for the presence of the presumed antecedent, this is logically referred to as a **case-control** study.

2. Equally, we could experiment by introducing a suspected "cause" (exposure) and then measure the subsequent effect in populations; this is called the **experimental epidemiology** approach. However, being limited by ethics and by the human situation, we often have to compromise rigor and simply observe the health effects of natural or social causes, such as war, immigration, population control, and changes in community policy on fluoridation. In these situations, as we discussed in the Introduction, it often is not possible for us as experimenters purposely to subject one part of the population to the exposure and leave the rest of the population free from exposure. Where we are unsure of the relative benefits of one or another exposure, experimentation may be possible. Examples of these would include testing whether one form of health service such as family practice is better than specialized care or whether one drug is better than another in treating selected diseases.

3. We could find groups with the presumed cause that were at that time *free* of the effect (health outcome) and then follow them over time to establish whether or not the expected effect is manifested. Thus, one is looking forward in time and doing a **prospective** study (from the Latin, *prospicere*, to look forward), also called a **cohort** study. In this instance, we would have as a control (comparison) group those who were also free of the effect but did *not* have the antecedent. They, too, would be followed over time to see if any of them manifested the effect.

Exercise 3.2

Many ideas about causal associations arise from the hunches of observant health workers of many professions, which eventually generate advances in epidemiological knowledge. Some such hunches heralded the sequence that established the causal relationship of cigarette smoking and cancer of the lung.

In 1927 Dr. F.E. Fylecote of Great Britain noted that in nearly every case of lung cancer he had seen or had known about, "the patient was a regular smoker, usually of cigarettes." In the United States, in 1936 Drs. Arkin and Wagner observed that of 135 men with lung cancer, 90% were "chronic smokers."

☐ a. What is different between these two statements of their impressions?

☐ b. What is missing from their observations that would be important for drawing conclusions?

Comment

a. Fylecote made no numerical judgment; he stated merely a hunch, no doubt over his cup of tea. The Americans, with their penchant for numbers, counted the smokers.

b. A control or comparison group is missing. In each instance, the researchers reported their hunches or observations about a group of cases. Often used in clinical studies, this approach is referred to as a **case-series** study. It often provides hunches for the epidemiologist to pursue.

In Britain "almost everyone," and *not only* lung cancer patients, could have been regular smokers. In the US, too, 90% of other sick people or 90% of everyone could have been "chronic smokers." Thus, smoking might not be associated with lung cancer specifically, but with being British, being sick, or being American. Nevertheless, these sorts of clinical anecdotal hints are important observations to be heeded and followed up in a more scientific manner.

You will know of other recent and important case reports and confirmatory studies of causes of diseases, which also started with astute clinical hunches. They include the association of diethylstilbestrol (DES) in pregnancy and cancer of the vagina in offspring, rubella in pregnancy, and congenital abnormalities, among many others.

Exercise 3.3

Often, the next step after clinical hunches in the epidemiological pursuit of causal association is a (retrospective) case-control study. It is frequently and easily carried out by health professionals in many settings.

☐ a. What are the steps in this case-control method?

☐ b. Why is the word "control" found in the name of this method?

☐ c. In what respects should cases be different from controls?

☐ d. In what respects should cases be similar to controls?

Comment

a. Find cases of the supposed effect (for example, disease) and obtain *from* them or *about* them the history of the assumed antecedent of cause (exposure).

Find control persons similar to the cases in those characteristics which are known to be related to the effect (potential confounders), such as age or sex but *without* the supposed effect, and similarly obtain histories of the exposure from or about them.

b. A control or comparison group is needed so that we can make sure that compared to noncases, cases had more of the exposure. Remember that epidemiology is a science of comparison of groups or aggregates. This is even more important in the case-control method, when the need for a comparison group is sometimes forgotten and only cases are studied.

c. Cases should differ from controls by having the health effect while the controls *do not* have the effect. This raises the importance of being able to decide what is a case and what is not a case. It sounds simple enough but many times there are as many opinions as there are people asked to define the health outcome. Think of some of the difficulties in defining some sorts of cases (for example, one who died, one who was dissatisfied with the medical care given, one who developed postoperative complications, one who developed schizophrenia). Try defining a case and then ask a friend to define a case. There may be considerable (and maybe even heated) discussion before you agree, if you ever do. Usually this problem is resolved by laying down objective criteria for identification of a case and applying them rigidly in the study.

d. Cases and controls should come from a similar population. The case-control study is one way the observational scientist tries to support causal associations by showing that people who developed the disease were similar to other people in the community *except* for the supposed antecedent. Thus, we are looking for differences in the frequency with which a supposed antecedent appears among the cases versus the controls. If our controls are chosen well, the *only* antecedent difference between cases and controls will be in the level of a characteristic that is related causally to the development of the disease. Using this comparison group strategy, we are controlling for many other characteristics that may confound our ability to show an association between a supposed antecedent and the disease. Hence, the use of the term "control" in case-control studies. This selection of controls is not easy and is never perfect, but there are ways of selecting controls that help us considerably in our comparisons.

In order to make our comparisons, we have to be able to gather "the evidence." Our investigation will certainly fail if we can only get information about the supposed antecedent for the cases and not for the controls, or vice versa. Thus, we must have access to information in a similar way for cases and controls and the quality of the information must be equally good for cases and controls.

The references given at the end of the chapter will guide you in selection of controls.

Exercise 3.4

In 1939 F.H. Müller carried out a case-control study in Germany; his findings are presented in Table 3.1.

Table 3.1 **Smoking Histories of Lung Cancer Patients and of Healthy Men of the Same Age, Germany, 1939**

		% of Group		
Group	Number	Heavy	Intermediate	None
Male patients with cancer of the lung	86	65.1	31.4	3.5
Healthy men of the same age group	86	36.0	47.7	16.3

Source: Adapted from: Doll R and Hill AB: *Brit Med J* 739–748, 1950.

Judging from the table, which of the following statements are correct? Give your thoughts on each.

☐ a. Smoking is associated with lung cancer, as shown by the fact that 65.1% of heavy smokers had cancer and only 36% were healthy.

☐ b. Smoking is associated with lung cancer as shown by the fact that 65.1% of lung cancer patients were heavy smokers and only 36.0% of healthy men were heavy smokers.

☐ c. The differences in rates are due to age differences, and the association between smoking and lung cancer is artifactual (that is, age is confounding the findings in Table 3.1).

Comment

We hope you read the title of Table 3.1. You can see that the members of the control group were of same sex and age as cases but did not have lung cancer.

a. 65.1 is the rate of heavy smoking in lung cancer patients and *not* the rate of lung cancer in heavy smokers. This is obvious because the rows and not the columns add to 100%. Similarly, 36.0% is the rate of heavy smoking in healthy men, and not the percentage of heavy smokers who were healthy. In a case-control study, we start with information about the health outcome (here, it is cancer) and look retrospectively in time at the extent of smoking (presumed antecedent) among cases and controls to see if this helps explain why the cases got lung cancer and the controls did not.

b. This statement is correct. But remember that if Müller's data are based on a sample from a larger population, which is usually the case, a test of significance must be done to see whether 65.1% and 36.0% differ (1) because of sampling variability or (2) because smoking behavior actually differs in the two populations of male lung cancer patients and healthy males. Let us assume that we have done the test of significance (it would be an χ^2 test, for those of you who may know some biostatistics) and have concluded that 65.1% and 36.0% "differ significantly"—the difference cannot be explained only by sampling variability.

c. No. We all know that age is related to smoking histories and that age *is* related to cancer of the lung, but the controls were "of the same age group" as the cases. Hence, age as a confounding variable was avoided in the selection of controls and cases by "matching" the two groups on age. Known associations with the disease under study are the bases of matching the cases and controls.

In matching, we try to control for confounding variables. If we do *not* match on a confounding variable, we can deal with it by eliminating it via subject selection, for example, by studying only males to eliminate sex as a confounding variable. Another way is through data analysis, as in adjustment of rates discussed in Chapter 1.

If you match on any characteristic, the cases and controls will be similar in that respect, so obviously one never matches on the antecedent (characteristic) to be tested.

Matching sounds easier than it really is. The more variables to be matched, the greater the universe we need from which to draw control patients. The problem is that if one is matching on age, sex, and social class, the control person has to be similar to the case on all three characteristics, not just on two or one. Homogeneous "captive" populations such as students or army inductees are always excellent matching sources, but they are relatively uncommon and not relevant to the study of many diseases. If you disagree about the difficulty of matching, select any five people and try to match them with other persons on, say five characteristics—and good luck!

For a more detailed explanation of matching, see the references at the end of this chapter.

Exercise 3.5

A later case-control study was carried out by Robert Schrek and others in 1950 in the United States. Their findings are shown in Table 3.2.

Table 3.2   **Smoking Histories in Male Patients
and Controls, USA, 1950**

Group	Total	% Nonsmokers
Male lung cancer patients*	82	14.6
Male patients with cancer of sites other than the lungs, larynx and pharynx, and lips*	522	23.9

*The distributions of age in these two groups were similar.

Source: Adapted from Schrek R, Baker L, Ballard G et al., *Cancer Research*, 10:49-58, 1950.

☐ a. Why did they select this sort of control population instead of healthy persons?

☐ b. Can the difference in the percentage of nonsmokers be due to the greater number of subjects (522) in the control population? Why or why not?

☐ c. What are the numerators and denominators for the rates in Table 3.2?

☐ d. In retrospective case-control studies, which is the characteristic or variable in the denominator, the disease being studied or the presumed antecedent (cause or exposure)?

☐ e. Which is in the numerator?

☐ f. Display Table 3.2 in a flow diagram, including the numbers in the respective boxes or positions.

☐ g. How could incorrect or biased reporting account for the difference in the percentage of nonsmokers?

□ h. What forces of selection might produce these findings?

Comment

a. The control group was chosen to see whether smoking histories are associated with all cancers or only cancer of the lung. Such control groups are often chosen on the basis of the *same* pathology in *different* sites to separate out site (local) specificity of cause and effect, or on the basis of *different* pathologies in the *same* site to separate out specificity of pathology. In this instance, a control group of noncancerous tumors of the lungs or chronic bronchitis cases would be examples of the latter sort of control group. Choosing the comparison group from patients admitted to the same hospital also minimizes the selective differences that bring people into the particular hospital.

Frequently a third control group of matched healthy persons is included to give the "baseline" comparison group for smoking (or nonsmoking) histories among nondiseased controls.

b. No, the percentages are rates.

c. In each instance, the numerator is the number of subjects in the nonsmoking category. The denominator is either the number of lung cancer patients (82) or the number of patients with cancer of sites other than upper respiratory and digestive tract (522).

d. and e. In all case-control studies, the item being looked at is the antecedent characteristic, and it must be in the numerator. We want to know, in effect, the rate of the "antecedent" in cases and controls. Therefore, numbers of cases and controls are the denominators.

f. Note, as shown in Figure 3.1, that in case-control studies subjects begin with the classification as "case" or "noncase" (control).

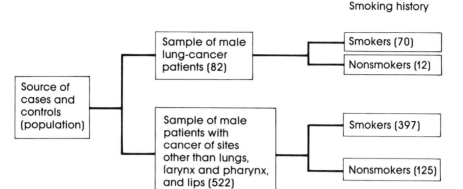

Figure 3.1 Smoking histories in male patients and controls, United States, 1950.

g. Having cancer of the lung may make patients overreport smoking (due to guilt, knowledge, selective memory). Having cancer of other sites, or being healthy, may produce underreporting because of nonconcern with remembering smoking or belief in a nonassociation. There would be biased reporting of the antecedent where the bias is produced by the disease (or effect).

h. Case-control studies are usually carried out on patients attending treament facilities as subjects. Those who are selected into the particular facility might differ from controls on some variables (for example, too poor to buy cigarettes, or live in an air-polluted industrial section of town). For this reason, controls may be chosen from admissions to the same facility. They then may share some of the same characteristics as cases attending the facility.

As in point prevalence studies, case-control studies include only those cases who have survived to that time. Thus, if cases who never smoked died more quickly than those who did smoke, there will be more cases around who smoked. This is another example of the selective survival concept. So case-control studies are only a variation of point prevalence studies with which they share many common weaknesses. This would not apply if one is doing a case-(incident-)control study using new cases, which requires that the time of manifestation of the effect be known. This can be ascertained from clinical records if the date of onset is known and recorded or by waiting for new cases to appear and then getting the history of their exposures to the possible "cause."

Exercise 3.6

☐ a. Using the flow diagram you constructed in Exercise 3.5, part (f), construct your own table showing the association of smoking history with lung cancer.

☐ b. Is there an association of smoking and lung cancer in this group? Why?

☐ c. From these data can you conclude that smoking causes lung cancer? Why?

Comment

a. Table 3.3, showing the association of smoking history and lung cancer, gives the number of cases and controls who were smokers and nonsmokers.

Table 3.3 **Distribution of Smoking History Among Male Cases of Lung Cancer and Controls, US, 1950**

Smoking history	Case	Control	Total
Smoker	70	397	467
	(85.4%)	(76.1%)	
Nonsmoker	12	125	137
	(14.6%)	(23.9%)	___
Total	82	522	604

Check to be sure you included the essential ingredients of a table—title (who, what, where, when), labels, column totals, and so forth. Note the direction of the percentages, with denominators being number of cases and number of controls.

b. Yes, 85.4% of lung cancer cases were smokers while 76.1% of the controls were smokers. Since cases and controls were exposed unequally to smoking, with *more* cases exposed, this may help to support the hypothesis of an association between smoking and lung cancer.

However, your answer should be tempered somewhat by your previous learning of the importance of sampling variability to the interpretation of this difference. A statistical test of significance will tell you the likelihood of sampling variability alone creating the observed differences between these sample rates.

c. This is a case-control or retrospective study. That is, we have information about the disease state (lung cancer) and are looking backward in time for evidence of differences between cases and controls in the antecedent or supposed cause (smoking). The problem is, however, that we do not know if the cases developed lung cancer and then started smoking or whether smoking started before their lung cancer. That is, we are unable to establish antecedent-consequent (cause-effect) relationships from the case-control study.

However, we are eager to quantify the risk of getting lung cancer among smokers, compared with (relative to) nonsmokers. The optimal way to obtain this is obviously to start with smokers and nonsmokers *before* they have cancer of the lung and then quantify the ratio of the rate of occurrence of new cases of lung cancer in these groups. This ratio (called the *relative risk*) is best derived from the optimal method described earlier. Exercise 3.7 will address this method, called a cohort or prospective study. However, if the study is a case-incident control one, and the date of onset of the effect is known, then estimates of the time relationship between effect and exposure are better. In this event, controls must have been selected as free from the disease (effect) at the time the new case is manifested.

Exercise 3.7

There is a technique for estimating this relative risk even though the data were derived from a case-control study. This estimate is called the odds ratio or the relative odds, which will remind you that it was derived from a case-control study. The technique has a solid mathematical base and is frequently used in case-control studies.

    ☐ a. From Table 3.4, assuming that we *know* that smoking preceded the occurrence of lung cancer (data are from a cohort study), what is the rate of lung cancer in smokers?

Table 3.4   **Frequency of Cases and Controls, by Smoking History**

Smoking history	Case	Control	Total
Smoker	a	b	$a + b$
Nonsmoker	c	d	$c + d$
Total	$a + c$	$b + d$	$a+b+c+d$

☐ b. What is the rate of lung cancer in nonsmokers?

☐ c. What is the ratio of the rate for smokers to the rate for non-smokers?

☐ d. If the disease is rare, then $a/(a+b)$ is approximately equal to a/b since a will be very small relative to b. Likewise, $c/(c+d)$ is approximately equal to c/d. If the disease is rare, how can the formula in part (c) be simplified for a cohort study?

☐ e. Apply the formula in part (d) to the case-control study in Table 3.3 in order to calculate the relative odds of lung cancer among smokers.

Comment

a. The rate is $a/(a + b)$ in smokers.
b. The rate is $c/(c + d)$ in nonsmokers.
c. The ratio is

$$\frac{a/(a + b)}{c/(c + d)} \quad \text{or} \quad \frac{a}{(a + b)} \times \frac{(c + d)}{c}$$

d. By assuming that $(a + b)$ is approximately equal to b and $(c + d)$ is approximately equal to d, the formula in (c) for a cohort study is simplified to $(a/b)/(c/d)$ or $(ad)/(bc)$. This formula seems easy to remember and is frequently used, so make sure you grasp it before proceeding.

As a reminder, this relative odds calculation will estimate the relative risk in a case-control study *if:* (1) the disease is relatively rare (there is difference of opinion among epidemiologists on how crucial this assumption is and/or how low the prevalence rate must be to qualify a disease as rare) and (2) cases included in the study are representative of all cases and controls are representative of noncases. Note that the controls may *not* be representative of the noncases if they have been matched with the cases.

e. $\dfrac{\text{Relative odds}}{\text{(odds ratio)}} = \dfrac{ad}{bc} \dfrac{(70)}{(397)} \dfrac{(125)}{(12)} = 1.84$

This means that in 1950 smokers in the United States had a risk of lung cancer 1.84 times the risk for nonsmokers. Further reading about the methods of estimating relative risks in case-control studies and the supporting assumptions can be found in the references to this chapter. Methods are also available for calculating a confidence interval around the risk estimate. A "confidence interval" is a statistical method to determine in what ranges of values the true risk is likely to be.

Exercise 3.8

☐ What are the advantages and disadvantages of the retrospective or case-control method?
Advantages:

Disadvantages:

Comment

Advantages of Case-Control Method

1. Cases are easily available. Thus, this is the method of choice in less common (rare) conditions and for studies done in clinical situations as opposed to community situations.

2. As with the prevalence (cross-sectional) option, it is quick and cheap and can be done by an interested person with access to clinical facilities.

3. It tends to support, but not prove, causal hypotheses by establishing associations.

4. Historical data are often available from clinical records of patients, so it is possible to do secondary analyses (analyses of existing data) without ever having to obtain further information from the cases or controls themselves.

5. The number of subjects needed to test the hypothesis of association is small compared to a cross-sectional design or a cohort design.

Disadvantages of Case-Control Method

1. Information regarding the antecedent is often dependent on memory and hence is potentially biased. Also, data from clinical records may be inadequate.

2. Criteria used in the diagnoses of cases may not be the same among doctors or researchers, so that "case groups" may not be homogeneous.

3. The chosen cases are selective survivors. The histories of the deceased cases may be selectively different from the cases who survive to be in the study, and we would never know it. Thus, the cases at one point in time do not represent a universe of cases. Nonrepresentativeness of cases also occurs because often hospital or clinic cases are used in studies, and these cases may be selectively different from cases who have not presented themselves for treatment, or from cases who went to a different facility. This restricts the generalizability of the findings to other populations. Making such generalizations from hospital or clinic samples to the general population may well be erroneous. Such a fallacy is called **Berkson's fallacy** after the statistician who first pointed it out.

4. The occurrence of the assumed antecedent in the history is obtained from selected cases and controls. Thus, the "antecedents" are not obtained from a universe of all antecedents, so we cannot know what the association would be on all or a representative sample of all people having the antecedent.

Exercise 3.9

☐ With so many seeming weaknesses, why and when does one choose the case-control method?

Comment

The case-control method is used often because it is easy, quick, and permits many health workers to test their hunches. It is done in select clinical or other similar situations, when the disease is rare, or when one does not have time, money, or inclination to launch a community study or long-term follow-up study.

We hope this urges you to follow up on your hunches—and to recall, when you are in doubt, that no hypothesis or hunch is ever wrong until disproven. Any hunches you or others develop are worth pursuing scientifically. Many great theories and discoveries were established by alert observers who, having hunches, tested them with facts, often in the face of bitter condemnation of their peers.

The essence of the epidemiological approach is one of the comparison of groups; thus, we use cases and controls. Many hunches are derived by astute and observant clinicians who only observe cases. It is very common to find descriptions of a group of cases without mention of a comparison group free of the disease. This approach is called a **case series approach,** which is not epidemiologic since there is no comparison group.

The choice of an appropriate comparison (control) group and its size is debated. Currently it is recommended that, where possible, four control subjects should be used for each case. This number will give maximal benefit in the analysis; more would be redundant, and less than four would be less powerful.

Summary

Here are the points you covered in Chapter 3. Check your understanding of them before proceeding to the next chapter.

1. The case-control study method.

2. The purpose of the control group and types of control groups.

3. Control of variables by sampling or by matching at the design stage.

4. Control of variables by analysis.

5. Calculation of relative risk estimates (odds ratio) from a case-control study.

6. Advantages and disadvantages of the case-control method.

References and Further Reading Sources

Topic	Reference number	Pages
Case-control method	16	279–284
	24	197–205
	27	103–121
	31	68–96
	36	191–225
	38	241–251
	40	314–316
	68	71–85
Odds ratio (relative risk from case control studies)	24	205–209
	36	209–216
	38	268–277
	40	316–321
Selecting controls and matching	1	33–38
	8	(article)
	9	(article)
	24	186–196
	38	244–256
	44	(article)
	68	115–124
Confidence intervals around odds ratio estimates	36	333–338
Berkson's fallacy	7	(article)
	11	(article)
	16	305–309
	39	(article)
	49	(article)

Cohort or Incidence Study Method: Looking Forward

4

In the earlier chapters, two epidemiological study strategies were introduced: the prevalence or cross-sectional method and the case-control or retrospective method. The cross-sectional study was a "snapshot" view of a representative sample or total population of a community in order to determine concurrent associations of a health condition and other group characteristics. The case-control study started with a determination of the health state (or condition) and looked backward in time (retrospectively) for the history of the presumed antecedent characteristic. In each of these study designs, associations may be supported but the antecedent-consequent relationship cannot be confirmed. Both designs fail to establish that the hypothesized cause (characteristic or risk factor) precedes the development or at least appearance of the effect (condition or health outcome).

The cohort method meets the need to confirm the causal association, the definite time/entity relationship missing in cross-sectional or case-control methods. It establishes time (secular) relationships between presumed antecedents and presumed effects, and in so doing, ensures knowing which came first. It is the method par excellence of epidemiological predictions and prognoses, for it can determine best the magnitude of risks for future events in those groups with specified characteristics. In establishing future outcomes, it thus provides health services with the knowledge about what antecedents to alter in order to prevent disease or promote health and the amount of reduction of disease such action can be expected to produce. Clearly, such a contribution is important in planning and evaluating any program related to the prevention of disease or complications of disease.

This method is the most potent available for use in analytic epidemiology. As opposed to retrospective techniques, the cohort method is referred to as a prospective (looking forward) strategy. In this instance, we can more directly identify those characteristics of groups or environments which are associated with a high risk or probability of future health events.

Health planners and administrators can capitalize on these findings in terms of predicting future health needs by knowing which characteristics precede disease. Cohort or prospective studies do confirm risk (or causal) factors and so present health promoters and educators with the health characteristics or behaviors that need modifying in order to prevent illness in society.

Exercise 4.1

☐ What are the logical steps in such a cohort (prospective, longitudinal, or incidence) study?

Write down your answer, then read the discussion below.

Comment

One starts with persons possessing the presumed cause (antecedent or exposure) *but free from the effect* (disease) and then waits for them to develop the effect. The comparison group (which is central to epidemiology) clearly must also be a group of persons who are free from the disease to start, but who in addition do *not* possess the presumed cause. These persons are watched for the same period of time to see if the new disease or effect develops.

In both groups, we await "new" effects or cases or incidents, for we are sure these events were not manifest at the beginning of the study. This permits us to call this, logically, the prospective, incidence, or cohort study method.

A cohort is very simply a group or aggregate of persons who have presumed antecedent characteristics in common and who are followed throughout their experience so that we may observe the development or nondevelopment of a given health outcome. Examples of a cohort might include: all new employees to a factory during a certain year, all the gall-bladder patients who were operated on in a given hospital during a certain period of time, or all the first-year students in a university during a certain year. The essence of a cohort study is (1) being able to define who is in the group and who is not and (2) putting some time bounds on the period (for example, what years) we are considering in observing our group or cohort of interest. The additional consideration epidemiologists require for a cohort to be used in an incidence study is that all the members of the group to be followed for a period of time are free of the health outcome at the start of the follow-up period. Only in this way can we look for "new" cases or incident cases of the health outcome of interest.

Exercise 4.2

☐ How does one ascertain those who are free from the disease (effect) at the beginning, and therefore at risk of becoming new cases or new events in the future?

Comment

In the beginning, we have to examine all persons in our sample or population and find out who has, or does not have, the effect and also the presumed antecedent. We then "forget about" (epidemiologically speaking, of course) those with the disease (effect), for they are no longer at risk of becoming a *new* event over time—they are "old events," already manifest. We confine our future prospective study to those free from the disease or health outcome under study.

Clearly, one has to be free of something in order to be at risk of becoming a *new* something in the future. An exception is being at risk of repeated episodes. Simply put, a person is only at risk of a first stroke if he has never had a previous stroke. But obviously he must have had his first stroke to be eligible for a second one. And the antecedents of the first stroke may be different from the antecedents of a second one.

Exercise 4.3

☐ In doing the initial assessment, what epidemiological method are we actually using?

Comment

We are actually carrying out a point prevalence or cross-sectional study. An incidence or prospective study always starts with a prevalence study to identify noncases and cases in the study population, and to ascertain the presence or absence of the antecedent that we're studying.

Exercise 4.4

☐ How do we calculate rates of the new events, that is, the incidence rates?

Comment

The numerator is the number of new cases or incidents over a time period. The denominator is the PAR (population at risk), *those free* from the disease or event at the start. Multiply by the usual constant (say 1,000) and express the rate per 1,000 persons per time period. Often the period is one calendar year, but this is arbitrary. One can express the rate for four-year or eight-year periods, or one can collect the new events over a number of years and express the rate as an average annual incidence rate. However, rates may change over time, so the longer the time period used, the more likely that we are putting together different rates into the average. In so doing, we may mask important secular variations (changes over time) in the rates or even the change in relationship of antecedent to effect. Obviously the longer the period covered by the rate, the greater its magnitude is likely to be. Thus, in comparing incidence rates resulting from different studies, do ensure that the time periods being compared are the same, or that average annual rates are used. This technique "neutralizes" the different periods. However, the relationship of incidence to time often is not linear because of an increase in the rates as time goes by and the cohort gets older. A note on terminology: such an incidence rate, called the **cumulative incidence,** is applied to a group of persons followed over the same period of time.

This will contrast with studies in which people are followed for different lengths of time (some drop out, or some come into the study at different times). In these, the denominator will *not* be the number of people, but rather the accumulated periods of time each person is in the study, that is, person years. The term **incidence density** is sometimes applied to such an incidence rate.

Exercise 4.5

☐ How does incidence differ from prevalence?

Comment

In the cross-sectional (prevalence) study design, we looked at a population or group and counted the number of persons in the group who had the disease at the time of the prevalence study. Those persons already had the disease and were available for counting or enumerating. Thus, the prevalence rate (PR) is

$$PR = \frac{\text{Existing cases}}{\begin{array}{c}\text{Persons eligible or "at risk" of being a case}\\ \text{(size of sample or population)}\end{array}} \times \text{Constant}$$

Incidence, however, establishes that everyone in the group who is eligible to develop the disease is also free of the disease at the beginning of the incidence study. Thus, the incidence rate (IR) measures the frequency of developing new cases.

$$IR = \frac{\text{New cases over a given time period}}{\begin{array}{c}\text{Persons at risk of becoming a new case}\\ \text{(free of the disease at the start of the study)}\end{array}} \times \text{Constant}$$

To review, when we begin our cohort study, we start with a cross-sectional study of a community or a sample from that community. The cohort of interest is those persons who are free of the disease at the start of the study and thus eligible to become new cases. This may be diagrammed as shown in Figure 4.1.

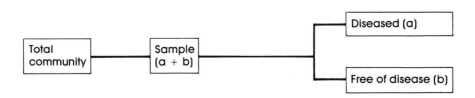

Figure 4.1 Finding the cohort.

The prevalence rate, PR, would be $a/(a + b)$. The cohort for use in the prospective study would be b, who would be followed into the future.

Exercise 4.6

The following is a hypothetical cohort study of coronary heart disease (CHD). In 1970, 1,000 men aged 30 to 59 years were examined. Of those, 50 had detectable CHD. Of those free from CHD in 1970, 64 developed CHD during the period 1971–1978.

☐ a. Calculate the point prevalence rate of CHD in 1970.

☐ b. Calculate the eight-year incidence rate of CHD for 1971–1978.

☐ c. Does this tell us the probability (risk) of development of CHD among males aged 30 to 59 over the eight-year period?

☐ d. If there were no deaths, no cures, and no migration between 1970 and 1978, what would the point prevalence rate be in 1978? (Steady on this one.)

Comment

a. A flow diagram like that presented in Figure 4.2 clearly shows the chain of events.

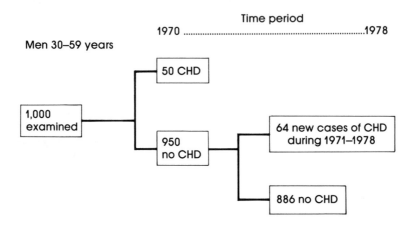

Figure 4.2 Cohort study of CHD, men 30–59 years.

The point prevalence rate of CHD in 1970 is 50/1,000, or 50 per 1,000 men 30 to 59 years old.

b. The eight-year (cumulative) incidence rate of CHD is

$$\frac{\text{New cases of CHD during 1971–1978}}{\text{PAR}}$$

This PAR *must be free* from the disease at the beginning of the time interval, so PAR = 950, *not* 1,000 men 30 to 59 years old. Those 50 CHD cases found in 1970 are not at risk of becoming *new* cases—they already have it!

Hence, the eight-year incidence rate of CHD is 64/950 × 1,000 or 67.4 per 1,000 men 30 to 59 years old. In the flow diagram, note that in each case the PAR or denominator is in the part of the diagram from which the numerator flows.

c. Yes. It is a probability (risk or likelihood) statement for men aged 30 to 59 in 1970 for the following eight years.

d. This is a sneaky question for the unwary beginner.

$$\text{PR in 1978} = \frac{\text{All cases of CHD prevalent in 1978}}{\text{PAR in 1978}}$$

$$= \frac{64 \text{ new cases and } 50 \text{ old cases}}{1,000} = \frac{114}{1,000}$$

or 114 per 1,000 men 38–67 years old (they are 8 years older).

The population remains steady at 1,000 because there were no deaths or migration. The numerator is all cases around in 1978, and with no deaths, cures, or migration of cases, it must equal 64 plus 50.

It is possible but unlikely to find during eight years that none of a population will migrate and that all the cases will survive for that period. This example does reinforce the point, however, that prevalence represents an accumulation of cases that survived, regardless of time of occurrence. In contrast, incidence rates pertain only to *new* cases during some time interval among a population initially free of disease.

Exercise 4.7

In assessing serum cholesterol as a cause (risk factor) of CHD, a cohort study carried out in Framingham, Massachusetts produced the results shown in Table 4.1. (Figures are approximated for ease of calculation in this exercise.)

Table 4.1   **Coronary Heart Disease Cases, White Men, Age 30–59, Framingham, 1950 and 1951–1958, by Levels of Cholesterol**

Serum cholesterol level (1950)	Population	CHD cases 1950	New CHD cases 1951–1958
Low cholesterol	1,120	20	66
High cholesterol	1,127	27	135
Total	2,247	47	201

Source: Adapted from the Framingham study. Kannel W, Dawder T, Kagan A et al., *Ann of Int Med* 55:33–50, 1961.

For each of the two cholesterol categories, do the following exercises.

☐ a. Calculate the prevalence rate of CHD in 1950 and the eight-year incidence rate of CHD for 1951–1958. Display them correctly in a table.

☐ b. Compare the differences between rates and comment upon the associations those rates have with cholesterol.

☐ c. Why is the denominator for the incidence rate in the high cholesterol *not* 1,120?

☐ d. Draw a flow diagram showing the logical progression of the study and the appropriate numbers in each classification.

Comment

a. Read the table heading.

Note that the age category is limited, but the wide age range may lead to age-related problems in analysis and interpretation within this age category. If all or most people with low cholesterol are 30 to 40 years old, and all or most people with high cholesterol are 41 to 59, and we do know that age is related to CHD, then any differences found between cholesteol categories may be due to age differences. Solution? Adjust for age or use smaller age categories or see whether our suppositions about age distribution within the cholesterol categories are correct, that is, whether age is an actual confounding variable in this study. Because the study considered only White men, any generalizations to other populations are restricted. Nothing can be said about females, Blacks, old or young people, Southerners, Bostonians, and so forth.

Table 4.2   *Prevalence Rates per 1,000 in 1950, and Incidence Rates per 1,000, 1951–1958, of Coronary Heart Disease, by Levels of Cholesterol Among White Men Aged 30–59, Framingham*

	Prevalence rate of CHD (1950)			Incidence rate of CHD (1951–1958)		
	Popula-tion	Cases	Rate	Popula-tion	Cases	Rate
Low cholesterol	1,120	20	17.9	1,100	66	60.0
High cholesterol	1,127	27	24.0	1,100	135	122.7
Total	2,247	47	20.9	2,200	201	91.4

Your table should look somewhat like Table 4.2. Make sure your table has totals.

b. The prevalence rate (PR) is slightly higher in the high cholesterol category than in the low category. The incidence rate is twice as great in the high cholesterol category as in the low category. Remember, though, if the data are based on a *sample* from a larger population, then a test of significance needs to be done before we can conclude that the larger rate for the high cholesterol group is not due merely to sampling variability (or, as some researchers would say, not due merely to chance). The smaller the size of the sample, however, the greater the sampling variability, and, therefore, the less the likelihood of finding differences to be significant (not due to chance). *Do not* assume automatically that differences are unimportant if they are *not* statistically significant. Conversely, statistically significant differences may have no real (biological) importance at all because it is possible to attain statistical significance simply by increasing sample size.

c. Because 20 of the population at risk had CHD in 1950 and are not at risk of being *new* cases, they are excluded from the PAR or denominator of the incidence rate.

d. Your flow diagram should resemble Figure 4.3. Note that in a cohort study, unlike in a case-control study, the sample is first differentiated on the basis of investigating the antecedent.

Flow diagrams are useful visual aids to thinking through a study; they help clarify the sources from which cases "flow." In each cholesterol category, the "new CHD" groups can only arise from the "no CHD" (free from CHD) categories of the 1950 prevalence study.

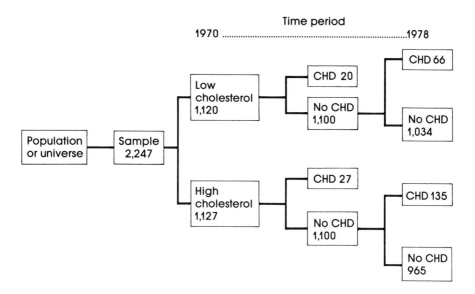

Figure 4.3 Cohort study of CHD, men 30–59 years.

Exercise 4.8

Because the study is prospective (remember, true cumulative incidence is calculated only from cohort studies), we can make risk assessments.

☐ Given the rates in Table 4.2, what is the relative risk for CHD of high cholesterol?

Comment

The **relative risk** is calculated by dividing the incidence rate in one group (those exposed) by the incidence rate in the other group (those not exposed): 122.7/60.0 = 2.04. As its name suggests, the ratio simply indicates relative degrees of risk. Thus, White men with high cholesterol in 1950 are 2.04 times more at risk of developing CHD than White men with low cholesterol. Clearly, in this study high cholesterol is associated as an antecedent with the probability of developing CHD.

The differences between the prevalence rates and incidence rates in Table 4.2 are also worth noting. Among the low cholesterol group, the incidence rate is about 3.5 times as great as the prevalence rate. However, this ratio jumps to 5.1 (122.7/24.0) among the high cholesterol group. The difference between the PR and the IR reflects the case fatality/cure rates. It can be assumed from these rates that the case fatality rate is higher among the high cholesterol group than among the low cholesterol group and probably that high cholesterol is a risk factor not only for becoming a case but also for dying from the disease. Or, perhaps the cure rate is larger in the low cholesterol group, but this is unlikely with CHD, which is not regarded as "curable."

Exercise 4.9

☐ How would you consider these incidence rates as indicators of the risks of developing the disease for *individuals* as opposed to groups?

Comment

In the low cholesterol group, the incidence rate is 60 per 1,000—out of every 1,000 White men aged 30 to 59 with low cholesterol, you could expect about 60 of them to develop CHD in an eight-year period. The probability, or chance, that a White man aged 30 to 59 with low cholesterol will develop CHD is 60/1,000 or 0.06 or 6 chances in 100. Naturally, the numerical value of any probability is always between zero and one.

This risk is a probability statement based upon this group's experience. If we were to apply this risk to a similar group of men over an eight-year period, we would expect approximately 6% of them to develop CHD or about 1% per year. But this does not allow us to identify *which particular* men will develop the disease, that is, whether the disease will occur in Mr. Jones's or Mr. Smith's heart.

Exercise 4.10

☐ How much greater was the risk in those with high cholesterol?

Comment

We repeat—*twice*, or more precisely $122.7/60 = 2.04$ times as great. Thus, using *relative risk*, we can say "the risk of a White man 30 to 59 years old in Framingham in 1950 developing CHD during the eight years 1951–1958 was 2.04 times greater for a man with high cholesterol as compared with a man with low cholesterol."

Exercise 4.11

Based on these data, it is logical to try and reduce cholesterol levels in all men to a "low" level in order to prevent new cases (incidence) of CHD.

☐ a. What would be the rate if everyone in the study had had low cholesterol?

☐ b. What reduction in the CHD rate would you get if you succeeded in lowering all the high cholesterol levels to low cholesterol levels?

□ c. Is this the amount of the risk you can attribute to being high in cholesterol?

□ d. How did we derive this risk assessment, and what do you call this risk?

□ e. By what proportion would we reduce the disease rate in the whole population if we successfully reduced all high cholesterol levels to low cholesterol levels?

Comment

a. The rate for the low category would be 60 per 1,000.

b. If IR_e is the incidence rate for the exposed group (high cholesterol) and IR_o is the incidence rate for the nonexposed group (low cholesterol), then $IR_e = 122.7$ per 1,000 and $IR_o = 60$ per 1,000. Therefore, expected reduction in the CHD rate is 122.7 minus 60 or 62.7 per 1,000 men with high cholesterol.

c. Yes.

d. We derived this risk assessment by *subtracting* the incidence rate in the low cholesterol (without risk or nonexposed) group from the incidence rate found in the high cholesterol (with risk or exposed) group. We call it the **attributable** (individual-based) **risk** (or risk difference)—which is what it is called by everyone in the field of epidemiology.

     e. A measure of the benefit in the population derived by modifying a risk factor is given as the **population attributable risk proportion,** also called *population attributable risk fraction.* This would be the proportion (or fraction) of the disease rate in *the whole population* that the rate in the exposed group represents. The total population rate minus the rate in the nonexposed group would be the amount contributed by the exposed persons, and that as a proportion of the total rate would give us the population attributable risk proportion (percent if multiplied by 100 or fraction if left as it is).

Exercise 4.12

☐ Calculate this population attributable risk percent (PARP) from the date in Table 4.2—it is fairly straightforward.

Comment

     The total population rate is 91.4 per 1,000. The rate in the nonexposed (low cholesterol) group is 60.0. Therefore, the *population attributable risk* is $91.4 - 60.0 = 31.4$ per 1,000. As you see, it is different from the simple (individual) *attributable risk,* which is $IR_e - IR_o$ or $122.7 - 60.0 = 62.7$.

     As a proportion of the total population rate, this population attributable risk is $31.4/91.4$ or $0.0314/0.0914 = 0.345$, or 34.5%.

Exercise 4.13

☐ Does this mean that 34.5% of the new cases of CHD in those Framingham men would be prevented if all had low cholesterol levels?

Comment

Yes, that is the meaning.

Exercise 4.14

☐ How could this help administrators, planners, and other health service people?

Comment

This population attributable risk percent (also called an etiologic fraction) does tell us what reduction in the disease or outcome (effect) variable we can expect if the exposure (risk factor) is removed. Because many diseases have more than one risk factor, we can calculate the PARP for each and weigh their relative values against the cost and feasibility of reducing or removing the risk and the reduction in cost that follows the reduction in the disease. Clearly, it can be used to evaluate a preventive program, too.

There are other methods for deriving this etiologic fraction (or population attributable risk percent), three of which we mention here for interest.

Method 1

1. Calculate the simple attributable risk (AR), $IR_e - IR_o$.

2. Multiply this by the prevalence (P) of the risk factor, $AR \times P = AR_P$ (or population attributable risk).

3. Divide this by the incidence rate of the disease in the total population (RT) or $(AR_P/RT) \times 100$, which equals the population attributable risk percent you calculated earlier. The mathematicians say they are equivalent; you can believe them.

Method 2

This method uses the relative risk (RR), which, you will recall, is IR_e/IR_o.

1. Multiply the prevalence of the risk factor (P) by (Relative Risk -1).

2. Divide this by the same entity $+ 1$, or

$$\frac{P(RR-1)}{P(RR-1) + 1} = PARP$$

You should try these formulae on the data and confirm that the same answer emerges. To nonmathematicians it is magic, but algebraically they are the same.

Method 2 using RR is most useful because we can derive estimates of relative risk from case-control studies in addition to cohort studies (you recall that we called it the odds ratio). We cannot truly get the attributable risk in such case-control studies, which makes method 2 applicable to both case-control and cohort studies.

Method 3

By subtracting the disease incidence rate in the nonexposed (IR_o) from the total rate of the disease (RT), a population attributable risk is established for that disease and that exposure in that population. The population attributable risk is $(RT - IR_o)$. To obtain a PARP, divide this difference by the rate in the total population (RT) and then multiply by 100. In brief, this method would be

$$PARP = \frac{(RT - IR_o)}{RT} \times 100$$

This is the method you actually used in Exercise 4.12. For further enlightenment, read the references given at the end of the chapter.

Exercise 4.15

☐ a. For review purposes, what does the relative risk tell us?

☐ b. What does the attributable risk tell us?

Comment

a. The relative risk tells us the ratio of the risk in one group or aggregate compared to the risk in another group. This ratio is useful to those in search of causative associations, but the size of the relative risk in no way indicates the magnitude of the incidence rates in the exposed and nonexposed groups. For example, a relative risk of 4.0 can be obtained from incidence rates for the following two diseases: (4 per million/1 per million) and (400 per 1,000/100 per 1,000). One disease is relatively rare, even in the exposed group, whereas the other disease is very common. You may decide that the rare disease affects so few people that no preventive action is warranted—even though the relative risk is 4.0.

However, relative risk does help to compare the relative contributions of risk factors no matter how much of the disease exists. Its size helps in deciding whether the association between the antecedent risk factor and the disease is a likely part of the causative web. Clearly if the relative risk is very large, regardless of the respective incidence rates, then a causative association is more likely.

b. The various measures of attributable risk (simple attributable risk, population attributable risk, and population attributable risk percent or proportion or fraction) all tell us in one way or another the amount of incidence of the disease that can be attributed to the antecedent cause. They can be used to estimate the *maximal* reduction of a disease rate in a community, if the antecedent (or exposure) is eliminated. We may have to eliminate many antecedents as more than one exposure is often involved in the causative network. Of course, the maximal reduction would be obtained only if everyone in the community had the antecedent and there were only one cause (antecedent). The smaller the percentage of community people who have the antecedent (the prevalence of the risk factor) and the smaller the risk attached to that antecedent, the smaller the reduction of the disease rate in the community produced by eliminating the antecedent. For that reason a highly prevalent risk factor (for example, smoking or hypertension) plus a high simple attributable risk (say, risk of lung cancer in heavy smokers or of heart disease and stroke in hypertensives) provides a large population attributable risk proportion, and thus a large potential reduction in these diseases.

Exercise 4.16

☐ What would influence the incidence or number of new cases?

Comment

Because incidence represents new cases, our answer must include whatever is associated with the development or prevention of new cases of the disease in question.

There are two main influences on incidence rates.

1. An increase in the proportion of the population who have the risk factors (antecedents, exposures) will raise the incidence. For example, if the blood pressure levels increase, stroke incidence will increase.

2. If preventive measures are known and being used, a decrease in their application will result in a rising incidence. For example, if immunization in children is cut down, the incidence of diphtheria and whooping cough will rise. Similarly, since the discovery and extended use of measles vaccine, we would expect the incidence of measles to decline.

In general, *treatment* of cases (cure or care) does not influence the incidence rate of the same disorder. Treatment of diseases occurs "after the horse is out of the barn," that is, treatment influences prevalence rates rather than incidence rates. Once a disease has appeared to warrant treatment, it is no longer possible to prevent it in that person. The exception, of course, is that treatment of a disease such as hypertension, which is a risk factor for stroke and coronary heart disease, may reduce the incidence rates of complications. But treatment of hypertension will not reduce the rate of occurrence of new cases of hypertension itself. This, in part, applies to infectious diseases also, for transmission is often effected before treatment is instituted. Similar considerations apply to chronic infectious diseases also.

Exercise 4.17

In a perfect cohort (incidence) study, which of the following will influence cumulative incidence rates? Check all correct answers and explain why or how.

☐ a. Immigration of cases into the study area.

□ b. Emigration of cases out of the study area.

□ c. Emigration of healthy persons out of the study area.

□ d. Immigration of healthy persons into the study area.

□ e. Changes in the case fatality ratio (proportion of cases dying).

☐ f. None of the above.

Comment

Only (f) is correct because in a cohort study the population *free* from the anticipated event is followed over time. Immigrants are disregarded since they are not part of the original cohort (study population). Emigrants from the original cohort are still followed over the time period to ascertain whether or not they manifest the event. A cross-sectional study, in contrast, will include immigrants if they arrive in time to be surveyed and exclude emigrants if they move the day before the survey.

Another technique, **life table analysis,** permits the entry of new people into the prospective study at different times, and permits them to be included in the study for different durations during the overall study period. Some may be in the study for one year, others for three years, and so forth. The denominator then becomes not *persons at risk* but *person-years* at risk after entrance into the study. The person-years approach has been an effective method of utilizing information on each member of the cohort, even if the period of follow-up of that person is short. As mentioned earlier, this is referred to as incidence density study. It is useful in that it uses all the data on participants in the follow-up study, even if they enter the study early or late. It still demands that persons on entry to the study be free from the effect (disease) and can be classified as to the exposure variable.

The life table analysis technique is another way of analyzing data from prospective or cohort studies. For further elaboration, read the references indicated at the end of this chapter.

Exercise 4.18

☐ List the advantages and disadvantages of the cohort study method. This one should be easy.

Advantages:

Disadvantages:

Comment

Advantages of the Cohort Study Method

1. It confirms causes because of the time sequence of the study.

2. Risk statements can be made, that is, the magnitude of the effect of the causative (risk) factor can be quantified.

3. It provides a baseline of rates of new cases against which preventive programs can be evaluated.

4. It provides planners with an estimate of the number of prevalent cases at the beginning point in the study. It also provides them with an estimate of the new cases that will require attention. Finally, it provides planners with the number and proportion of cases they can prevent if they are successful in reducing the risk factors.

5. It analytically tests hypotheses of cause and effect and enables an estimation of the relative contributions of different causes to the occurrence of the effect (disease or outcome).

6. It helps reduce factors of information bias. Selective recall/memory does not occur as a result of the disease or the health state already being manifested. Those responsible for classifying the subjects at the start cannot know who will eventually get the disease and so cannot consciously or unconsciously introduce information bias in categorizing the antecedent.

7. Bothersome selection factors are minimized because "disease-free" representative samples of a cohort with and without the presumed causal characteristics are followed over time. Thus, the incidence figures are not influenced selectively by the presence of the effect (outcome, disease) at the beginning of the study.

8. Selective migration of cases or of healthy subjects is not a problem because the original cohort is followed even if they migrate.

Disadvantages of the Cohort Study Method

1. The time required to achieve answers is longer for a prospective study, especially if the determination or latent period between the antecedent characteristic and the effect (outcome) is long.

2. Some participants leave the geographic area of the study and cannot be traced; some die with no known cause or lose interest in participating; some are inevitably "lost" to follow-up for the effect, despite intensive efforts to track them. This introduces selection bias.

3. Because of the time required, because of the effort involved in tracking down participants for follow-up, and because more than one examination of the subjects is required for the presence of the disease, this type of study is expensive.

4. Participation rates in cohort studies are lower than in cross-sectional studies for they require a longer time of cooperation by participants.

5. Unexpected changes in the environment or culture that occur during the follow-up period may influence the associations of the disease and the antecedent over time. It is usually hoped that these events or behaviors affect the comparison groups equally, but they may not. For example, participants may change their attendance for health care or their exposure to the antecedent (such as a nonsmoker beginning to smoke during the study period).

6. For diseases of relatively low incidence (there are many) this type of study is not feasible because none or very few persons in the sample may actually manifest the disease. Usually an estimate of the expected incidence is required before embarking on this effort. The investigators need to know how many cases can be expected among subgroups and how long they will need to follow them to get answers to the questions of association that they seek to address.

Exercise 4.19

☐ Does this mean, then, that an incidence or prospective study gives conclusive proof that the antecedent causes the health outcome?

Comment

Some people will say not, although admitting certainly that cohort studies give more evidence to support causal hypotheses than do cross-sectional or retrospective studies. There are still some people who maintain that all of the prospective studies on smoking and lung cancer do *not* prove that smoking causes lung cancer. They claim that a third factor exists somewhere, still undiscovered, that is confounded with both smoking and lung cancer. This third factor causes you to want to smoke and also causes you to get lung cancer. Hence, they claim, smoking per se is not at all related to lung cancer.

Of course, such an argument can be brought to bear on *any* prospective study, and there is always a chance that the argument is true. What you have to do in such a case is use your best judgment of all available scientific evidence to judge the plausibility of the argument.

There is also the practical consideration that preventive health care can be successful without knowing the absolute direct cause of a health problem. Consider that draining swamps can improve the malaria situation even without knowing that the mosquitoes living in the swamps are the real culprits.

The history of the epic studies in preventive medicine support this notion. John Snow associated cholera with polluted water years before Robert Koch identified the causative organism, James Lind prevented scurvy in sailors centuries before vitamin C was identified, and Goldberger associated pellagra with a corn diet before the vitamin B factor was identified. There are many others.

Later in this manual, we will consider the rules of evidence on the nature of associations. This is an important area for you to grasp so you can meet the challenges ahead in decision making, and it is not easy.

As an aside, the term "hybrid study" has been applied to a combination type of study. It would start as a case- (incident-) control study, with recording of the date of onset of the effect (case), with estimates of the exposure of both cases and controls (people free from the effect at the start of the study). The controls would then be followed up as in a cohort study with new cases being added to the previously recognized cases. The problems of this mixture are those which arise from case-control and cohort studies; the advantage is that it shortens the follow-up time necessary.

Exercise 4.20

We have guided your consideration of the differences in prevalence and incidence rates. It is quite possible to have both prevalence and incidence rates for a specific disorder. It is important that you know the inferences that are and are not possible from comparing these rates over time (the secular trends). Table 4.3 shows some hypothetical rates.

Table 4.3   *Prevalence and Incidence Rates per 1,000 (Hypothetical)*

Year	Prevalence rate (per 1,000)	Annual incidence rate (per 1,000)
1970	70	15
1980	71	8
1990	69	4
2000	70	1

☐ Compare the secular changes in these rates. What could produce these relative changes in rates?

Comment

In Table 4.3, the prevalence rate remains steady over time and the incidence rate declines. The proportionately fewer new cases may be due to a successful preventive program or to the antecedents of the disease disappearing or decreasing. But why is the PR steady during the same period?

Cases must be getting better care so that there is longer survival with the disease and lower death rates of cases. An increased cure ratio could not be occurring because that would cause the PR to decline.

Another possibility is that the cure ratio went up but was balanced by immigration of "old" cases who kept the PR steady but were not included as new cases in incidence.

Thus, the interplay of incidence and prevalence is related to the case fatality or case cure ratios—those forces which determine the presence of cases in the prevalence "pool." You should recall from Chapter 2 that prevalence varies with incidence and duration.

Exercise 4.21

Figure 4.4 consists of diagrammatic representations of four patterns of secular trends of point prevalence rates (PR) and incidence rates (IR).

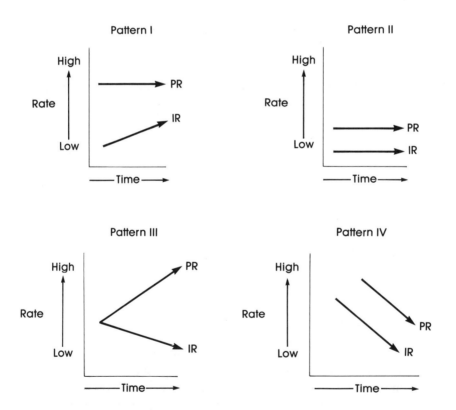

Figure 4.4 Different patterns of incidence and prevalence rates.

☐ Interpret each pattern, indicating possible explanations of each.

Comment

Pattern I

The incidence rate has increased over time, but the prevalence rate has remained steady. Possible explanations are that (1) the cure ratio might be improving and/or (2) the case fatality ratio might be increasing, so duration of disease is shortened. With such a secular increase in the incidence rate, the preventive program clearly is not too effective.

Pattern II

There is no change in either rate over time. Case cure and case fatality ratios must have been steady with no migration of either cases or healthy people.

Pattern III

Although the incidence rate has declined, the prevalence rate has increased. Perhaps the cure ratio has decreased over time, or the care has improved and thus more cases are surviving longer and are still available to be counted as cases. Thus, over time, the case fatality ratio has decreased.

In this pattern, either the preventive program is successful or else the antecedents are lessening, perhaps by migration of high risk persons, or the antecedents are not as harmful because of other changes, such as the development of immunity or resistance.

Pattern IV

Both incidence and prevalence have decreased. The declining incidence, again, may be due to diminishing occurrence of risk factors or to better prevention. The fact that prevalence has kept pace with it indicates that the case indices (death and cure ratios) have remained fairly constant.

This interplay among incidence, prevalence, and case fatality/cure ratios can be responsible for many different secular patterns. They are easy and intriguing to consider. Try some of your own design.

Exercise 4.22

Prevalence rates and incidence rates have importance in the evaluation of different aspects of health and medical care.

☐ To what service factors is each rate related, as an evaluative index?

Comment

In evaluation terms, the prevalence rate may reflect better or worse care and/or cure of cases since prevalence reflects the case load in the community. The incidence rate reflects the outcome of preventive programs since incidence estimates the introduction of new cases of the disease.

Exercise 4.23

Table 4.4   ***Ten-Year CHD Incidence Rates per 10,000***
White Men, Aged 30–59 at Entry, Framingham,
by Starting Cholesterol Level

	Cholesterol level			
	Low	Moderate	High	Very high
CHD incidence rate	514	708	914	1,553

Source: Same as for Table 4.1.

☐ Comment upon Table 4.4.

Comment

The higher the cholesterol level, the higher the incidence rate. The "very high" category has an exceptionally high CHD incidence rate. The relative risks for the "very high" category are approximately three times that for the "low" category, two times that for the "moderate" category, and 1.7 times that for the "high" category.

The likelihood of an association between a characteristic and a disease being causal is enhanced if a stronger "dose" or more of the antecedent produces higher rates, that is, a "dose-response" relationship is shown. Thus, the more cigarettes and the longer the time one smokes, the greater should be the risk of lung cancer.

The existence of a dose-response relationship between a risk factor and a disease is another finding that lends credence to associations being causal. A test of statistical significance will measure the probability of these differences in rates arising due only to sampling variability (or "chance"), but it does not address the possible causal nature of associations.

The finding of a dose-response relationship also supports the differences in rates as real reflections of population parameters that differ. Such logical incremental relationships are not likely to be due to sampling variability. Recall that the size of the sample and the amount of difference between the groups' rates (the parameters) influence the statistical test results. So these tests of significance are tools to assess only one element in our interpretation of these differences and not more than that.

Exercise 4.24

In the same prospective study, other risk factors such as definite hypertension and electrocardiographic (ECG) evidence of left ventricular hypertrophy (LVH) were identified.

Table 4.5   ***Six-Year Incidence of CHD per 1,000 White Men Aged 40–59, According to Combinations of Blood Pressure, Serum Cholesterol, and ECG Evidence of LVH at Initial Examination***

	Incidence rate
Normal on all three	36
Abnormal on only one	103
Abnormal on two only	204
Abnormal on all three	500

Source: Same as for Table 4.1.

□ Comment upon Table 4.5.

Comment

The incidence rate increased with the increasing number of risk (antecedent) factors, but not arithmetically (not steadily by a fixed amount). The risk for those who are abnormal on all three (500) is much greater than expected by simple addition of the risks for one (103) or two (204) abnormalities. This suggests some interaction of the factors, that the presence of one factor enhances the detrimental effects of the others.

Exercise 4.25

□ What does Table 4.5 indicate is the relative risk of CHD for White men aged 40 to 59 with all three risk characteristics compared with (a) those with two characteristics only and (b) those who were normal? What do these suggest?

Comment

a. RR = 500/204 = 2.4 times
b. RR = 500/36 = 14.0 times
The nonarithmetical increase in relative risk as the number of abnormal risk factors increases suggests interacting risk factors.

Exercise 4.26

We learned that one disadvantage of the cohort study method is the time it takes to wait for outcomes to happen. The well-publicized Framingham study lasted 20 years or more. As a way of avoiding this delay, what do you think of the possibility of having a cohort and its data available at some time in the past, information about their outcomes since, and the possibility of finding them *now* and seeing their status?

    ☐ a. Is this, in concept, the same as a cohort study started now?

    ☐ b. Under what circumstances can one do these cohort studies, starting in prevous times, but done now?

Comment

    a. Yes. It is a cohort studied over a period of time.

    b. Any time a cohort of persons can be identified who are known to be free of the health outcome of interest, on whom measures of the antecedent characteristic can be obtained, and who can be followed forward in their time, they can be utilized in a cohort study. When investigators do their research today on a cohort defined in the past, the study is similar to a cohort study even though the cohort was formed in the past. Just as with the usual cohort study (starting in the present), it requires persons to be free of the disease, to be stratified on the basis of the antecedent characteristic and followed forward in time. The period of follow-up may also have ended in the past (before the present), if data are available about the occurrence of new events over a period of time. The follow-up may also continue into the present or future.

Exercise 4.27

    ☐ Can you think of a reasonable name for such studies that would best identify their characteristics?

Comment

This study design has been given many names most of which confuse even the professional epidemiologist. The most useful name, we think, is a **historical cohort study.** For those with an interest in semantics, try out the other names for this study design: historical prospective study, retrospective prospective study (looking back, looking forward), reconstituted cohort study (like instant grits), retrospective cohort study, and noncurrent prospective study. Confused? You are not alone. We recommend that you remember the designation that best illustrates it for you.

Exercise 4.28

The historical cohort study has been widely used in studies in occupational settings where population registers (payroll records, for example) are available historically and medical records are accessible for the period of study follow-up.

☐ Can you think of other examples of available registries or data banks recorded in the past that could form the bases for historical cohort studies?

Comment

Most countries keep birth certificates for everyone, often prenatal records, examinations of school children or army inductees—all these may be available on past cohorts who could be ascertained now for likely outcomes. There are many others; for example, survivors of the atomic bomb explosions and their offspring are still being followed up. Children of mothers who took diethylstilbestral (DES) years ago during pregnancy also represent past cohorts available now.

Perhaps you know of other cohorts that possessed a characteristic years ago that is now relevant to today's health outcomes. Naturally, the rules of any scientific study apply, including standardized criteria for categorization of characteristics and outcomes, good reproducibility and validity of instruments and observers, and correct controls (comparison groups).

Cohort studies are the most powerful strategy we use in epidemiology. We hope you enjoyed learning about them.

Summary

The main points covered in this chapter include:

1. Following a cohort of healthy individuals forward in time and observing the incidence of disease among strata of the characteristic.

2. Relationship of incidence rate and prevalence rate.

3. Calculation, uses, and interpretation of

a. relative risk,

b. attributable risk, or simple attributable risk,

c. population attributable risk,

d. population attributable risk percent or population attributable fraction or etiologic fraction, and

e. estimates of community impact of programs.

4. Advantages and disadvantages of the cohort study design.

5. Historical cohort study method.

Comment

Yes, all of them. We could associate taking of certain medications with presence or absence of diseases at a point in time in a sample of a population (cross-sectional strategy). We certainly could get history of the drug taking or exposure to family versus specialty practices, from some persons with and others without the expected outcome (case-control method). We could follow through time from now on, or from a previous period if data are available, a cohort of persons free from the effect but having taken one or other medications, or having been exposed and not been exposed to the experimental factor, and see if there is a difference in the outcome that is conceptually linked to the event.

So it seems that we can apply all three strategies. In experimental epidemiology, though, the investigator often decides what the experimental factor will be and furthermore, which participants receive it and which participants do not. This type of research gives the investigator more control over the situation than in the case, for example, where participants themselves decide whether they have the antecedent or not (for example, smoke or not, use oral contraceptives or not, take a certain drug or not).

There are quasi-experimental (literally "as if experimental") situations in which the investigator does not have as much control as in the experimental situation as to who does or does not receive the experimental factor, for example, experiments of "nature" such as earthquakes or famines. These situations, however, do expose a large number of persons to some factor and give opportunities for epidemiological pursuits.

Many epidemiological observations of the health effects of natural occurrences have led astute observers to great results. These include the historical greats mentioned before: Snow on cholera (Her Majesty's anaesthesiologist doing epidemiology as a hobby); Gregg, an Australian opthalmologist, demonstrating the association of rubella in pregnancy with congenital abnormalities; and Goldberger, an American internist, proving the dietary cause of pellagra. There is a place for all of us who open our eyes and minds to observe nature at work.

Exercise 5.3

Usually, however, experimental epidemiology denotes an actual attempt to try out some drug or treatment or program on a group and compare their outcomes with a control group's experience without the intervention.

☐ How would one carry out such a trial of, for example, a new drug to treat cancer?

Comment

Treat a group of cancer patients with the drug and compare the group's survival or cure ratio with another group of similar cancer patients not given the same drug.

Exercise 5.4

Other considerations enter into our thoughts and consciences now.

☐ a. Is it ethical to experiment, and under what conditions?

☐ b. Can we have our control group take no treatment? And under what circumstances?

☐ c. Must we have a control group, or can we do a before and after trial? For example, can we see what the effect of a drug is on arthritic patients by comparing the severity of symptoms, such as pain, before and after the drug is taken? What are your thoughts on this issue?

Comment

a. The ethics of human experimentation is a difficult and important issue. It is ethical when there is no effective treatment and the new treatment has an acceptable chance (perhaps based upon animal experimentation) of success, *without* dangerous or severely unpleasant side effects. However, experimentation is not ethical when the treatment is hazardous and satisfactory treatments are available.

Sir Austin Hill in Chapter 1 of his book *Statistical Methods in Clinical and Preventive Medicine*[30] deals superbly with these considerations. He does state that it is sometimes unethical *not* to experiment, which makes sense, for all too often a new technique is popularized (such as coronary bypass surgery for coronary heart disease) before an adequate trial is carried out.

b. Yes, if and *only if* the withdrawal or withholding of all treatment is not detrimental to the life and well-being of subjects, and they are so informed. For example, withholding of treatment in an experimental trial of a new common cold treatment would be reasonable, or substituting a placebo in its place. (A *placebo* is a treatment that is believed by the investigator to have no effect but is believed by the subject to be an effective treatment. The word is derived from the

Latin, meaning "shall be pleasing.") Such withholding or placebo treatment would not be ethical if the disease were pneumonia. As a result, often the new treatment group's results are compared with the usual, or best available, treatment group's results.

c. The participant in a trial sometimes can be his or her own control by providing a before and after comparison. This applies especially in drug trials where the drug action is temporary and the individual inevitably returns to his or her original state later. In this case, drugs can be assessed for effects on a before and after basis. The advantage here is that the experimental variability is reduced. But there are few circumstances when these conditions pertain, for usually we want to see if a drug affects the natural history of an illness. A before and after trial using only an experimental group could be used to investigate prevention of motion sickness, alleviation of chronic symptoms of an unremitting nature, or change in some usually stable physiological measures. Further reading on the issue of "before and after" or "subject as his own control" is referenced at the end of this chapter.

Other aspects, such as cost, side effects, and clinical indications enter into deciding choice of treatments, but they are only partly epidemiological. It is therefore imperative that all participants, even volunteers, be fully informed prior to their written consent to participate in the trial.

In recent years, there has been increasing professional and public sensitivity to the issues involved in research with human participants—this is true for all types of study designs, not only those with some experimental element. In the effort to protect study participants, substantial local and federal guidelines have been drawn to regulate research activities. Because these regulations vary by locality and change rapidly over time, it is impossible to present them in a manual of this nature. Any of us, however, who plan to undertake an epidemiological or any other kind of study should be familiar with local and federal "human subjects" procedures pertinent to our efforts. It is important to remember that scientific progress in studying health of humans can only be made in a social context.

Where such guidelines do not exist, advice should be sought from professional and community leaders as to the acceptability of the intended trial and the conditions under which it can be carried out in the particular area or country.

Exercise 5.5

☐ Draw a schematic flow diagram outlining a clinical therapeutic (treatment) trial study.

Comment

The format, which is much the same as a prospective study, is well illustrated in Figure 5.1.

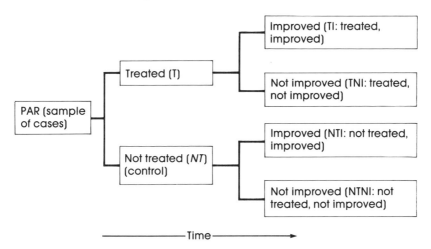

Figure 5.1 Flow diagram for an experimental epidemiological study.

Exercise 5.6

☐ For this clinical trial to be effective—to show that the treatment was effective—what rates would be compared and be different? Use the notations of the flow diagram.

Comment

For the treatment to be effective, the improvement rate in the treated group (TI/T) should be greater than the improvement rate in the untreated (NTI/NT), and the differences in rates should be unlikely to be due to chance (sampling variability).

Exercise 5.7

☐ As with other control groups, such as in case-control or cohort studies, the clinical trial requires its control group to possess certain characteristics. What are they? (This is fairly logical.)

Comment

The control group should be similar to the treatment group with respect to all characteristics that are associated with the expected outcome (recovery), but it should *not* receive the treatment under study.

As we mentioned earlier, the control group can sometimes be deprived of treatment or receive the usual treatment or receive a placebo. Placebos are given to "control" the nonbiological or nonpharmaceutical effect of the test treatment (for example, attention being paid to the subject). Note, however, that placebos may have an effect themselves. For further details, read references given at end of this chapter.

Exercise 5.8

☐ In which ways can such comparable control subjects be obtained?

Comment

A frequently used way is to take all participants eligible for the clinical trial according to the study criteria, for example, all males with third-stage prostatic cancer, and assign them to the treatment or control groups at random. This is called randomizing the allocation of subjects. Randomization should produce two or more groups similar on all characteristics not controlled via other methods such as subject selection.

Exercise 5.9

☐ What do you understand by random allocation?

Comment

Random allocation simply means that each subject has an equal chance of being assigned to any group. This can be done in many ways, ranging from simply tossing a coin to using a table of random numbers, found in many books of statistics. The researcher makes the decision of allocation to groups using some random scheme. Random allocation of subjects should be done whenever possible because it is an acceptable method for obtaining treatment and control groups that are comparable.

Random allocation can be used along *with* matching; for example, the researcher may match on race and sex. Then, for a pair of white females who are matched, the researcher would randomly assign one subject to the treatment group and one subject to the control group. Each matched pair would be randomly assigned to the two groups, which would then have the same sex and race distribution. They should have about the same distribution on other variables due to the random allocation of subjects.

Because of the frequent use of random allocation, the term "randomized clinical trial" or "randomized therapeutic trial" is used to describe this experimental epidemiology method. For further reading on randomization, see references at the end of the chapter.

Exercise 5.10

In the first clinical study to test the efficacy of streptomycin in the treatment of pulmonary tuberculosis, the results shown in Table 5.1 were found.

☐ a. Calculate the correct rates to establish whether streptomycin treatment is more effective than the control drug.

Table 5.1   ***Improvement Status by Radiological Assessment After Six Months Treatment of Similar Tuberculosis Patients Randomly Assigned to Streptomycin and Control Drug Treatment***

	With considerable improvement	Without considerable improvement	Total
Streptomycin	28	27	55
Control drug	4	48	52
Total	32	75	107

Source: Adapted from: Streptomycin treatment of pulmonary tuberculosis: A medical research council investigation. *Brit Med J* 2:771, 1948, Table II.

□ b. Draw a flow diagram to illustrate the above prospectively, putting the figures in the correct positions.

Comment

"Considerable improvement" rate in patients treated with streptomycin is 28/55 = 50.9%. "Considerable improvement" rate in patients on the control drug is 7.7%. Of course, we would need to do an appropriate test of significance to see if the two percentages 7.7% and 50.9% differ significantly. Because they do, streptomycin is more effective than the control drug. This analysis is done prospectively, as therapeutic (or clinical) trials are usually done. If you compared in the other direction—28/32 = 87.5% of those who were "considerably improved" had received streptomycin, as compared with only 27/75 or 36.4% of those without considerable improvement—you would be analyzing a prospective trial in a retrospective manner. Such inappropriate analysis of data seems to reduce the advantages of prospective versus retrospective strategies.

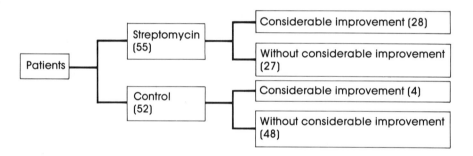

Figure 5.2 Flow diagram for study on effectiveness of streptomycin.

This form of a therapeutic trial has illustrated the epidemiological method applied in clinical situations as contrasted to entire populations or communities. It is one example of clinical epidemiology using the experimental approach. For further reading on clinical trials, see the references at the end of this chapter.

Exercise 5.11

What about a follow-up or prospective study of cases as opposed to a cohort of exposed people?

☐ a. Is this of value? Why?

☐ b. What sort of questions would it answer?

Comment

a. The case follow-up study is the descriptive epidemiology of the natural history of diseases and the risk of various outcomes of the diseases (such as complications). It documents many antecedents (risk factors or preventive factors) in the changing patterns of the course of the disease over time and also includes the epidemiology of recovery from disease.

b. It would tell us what influences natural remissions, deaths, changes in symptomatology, or other complications. These may not be the same factors as antecedents of the original disease.

To date, major risk factors for the initial attack or incident of myocardial infarction (MI or heart attacks) would include hypertension, cigarette smoking, personality type, and others. But the major risk or antecedent of *repeat* attacks of MI is a previous attack, with less evidence that the high risk characteristics for the first attack are as significant in the risk process of subsequent attacks. Thus, factors important in the first attack are not necessarily the same as those which lead to good rehabilitation from the illness or the likelihood of another attack. Controlling hypertension may well prevent the first attack of stroke but it may not necessarily reduce the risk of subsequent attacks. So establishing the antecedent of a disorder does not mean necessarily that removal of the risk (or antecedent) factor will necessarily reduce the rate of repeat attacks of the disease. This possibility needs testing to become a fact.

Exercise 5.12

☐ a. What is clinical epidemiology, apart from experimental epidemiology in the community?

☐ b. How does it relate to experimental epidemiology at the community level?

Comment

a. Clinical epidemiology embraces the study or knowledge of health states of groups or aggregates but is usually applied to available, chosen clinical patients only and therefore is selective. It includes the application of all the research design strategies—cross-sectional, retrospective, prospective—in the trial of treatments, description of the natural history of illness, or tests of preventive care.

b. It relates closely to community epidemiology. For example, antihypertensive drugs (those which lower blood pressure) were found, tested, and proven effective in therapeutic tests with selected hypertensive patients by the procedure of randomized clinical trials. Then, the population- or total community-oriented epidemiologist or other professional set out to test the treatment of *all* or a representative sample of hypertensives *in a community* and aimed to lower blood pressure and thereby reduce complications (strokes, deaths) in the sample of the *total* community. The hoped-for result is a reduction in

ware of her initial findings when doing the repeat examinations on each of the 30 specimens.

☐ Why was it so important that she did not know the result of her first examination when examining the same urine specimens for the second time?

Comment

Tests of reproducibility are of value only if each labeling or examination result for a given test is independent of the knowledge of previous examination results on that specimen or person. This is because knowledge of prior results can influence later labeling and thereby inflate the proportion of similar results on the two examinations. This is not necessarily intentional cheating but may be due to the human tendency to call things as we think or hope they should be, rather than as we see them. This tendency makes it important that we have no prior knowledge of the previous results in doing tests for reliability.

Exercise 6.3

Table 6.1 shows the hypothetical results of two independent examinations for the presence or absence of sugar done by one nurse on the *same* 30 specimens of urine. Results of the urine sugar tests were scored as negative (0), positive (+), or strongly positive (++).

Table 6.1   Amount of Sugar in Urine Specimen on Two Examinations

Urine specimen number	Exam 1	Exam 2	Urine specimen number	Exam 1	Exam 2
1	+	0	16	+	+
2	0	0	17	+ +	+ +
3	+ +	+	18	0	+
4	0	+	19	0	0
5	+ +	+ +	20	+ +	0
6	+	0	21	0	+ +
7	0	0	22	0	0
8	+ +	+	23	+ +	0
9	+	+	24	+	0
10	+	+ +	25	0	0
11	0	0	26	+	+ +
12	+	+	27	+ +	+
13	0	0	28	0	+ +
14	0	0	29	0	0
15	0	+ +	30	0	0

These data can be summarized by a frequency distribution for each examination, as shown in Table 6.2.

Table 6.2   Frequency Distribution of Amount of Sugar in Urine, by Examination

Amount of sugar	Exam 1	Exam 2
0	15	15
+	8	8
+ +	7	7
Total	30	30

□ Do these results tell us that her examinations are 100% reproducible? Why do you think that?

Comment

No. The identical frequencies in Table 6.2 for 0, +, and + + on the two examinations are misleading. The same totals can be, and in fact were, obtained even though different results were obtained for some specimens on the two examinations. Totals (or table marginals) never provide adequate information from which to judge reproducibility or reliability. We need to compare the results of the two examinations *for each specimen*, that is, we need to see for how many specimens the nurse got the same result on both examinations.

It is all very logical; one must keep alert, however, because sometimes reliability tests are reported giving only the totals. Do not be fooled: the comparison of two independent examinations may look very good, but unless it compares results for individual cases or specimens, it is not telling you what you need to know about reliability.

Exercise 6.4

☐ a. Put the results of the two examinations in a table to permit you to calculate the correct index of reproducibility.

□ b. How reproducible are her examinations? Express it as a percentage.

□ c. How good is that, and why do you think so?

Comment

a. Your table should look like Table 6.3. We hope you put in the title and headings.

Table 6.3 **Frequency Distribution of Amount of Sugar in 30 Urine Specimens, by Results of Two Examinations**

		Exam 1: amount of sugar			
		0	+	+ +	Total
Exam 2:	0	10	3	2	15
amount of	+	2	3	3	8
sugar	+ +	3	2	2	7
	Total	15	8	7	30

Just to make sure you understand the table, what does the number 3 mean in the first row of the table? It means that there were three specimens (out of the 30) for which the nurse gave a result of + on the first examination and 0 on the second examination.

b. Her reliability (reproducibility, repeatability) index is

$$\frac{10 + 3 + 2}{30} = \frac{15}{30} = 50\%$$

Note that we added the frequencies in the diagonal of the table.

c. Not very good. It indicates that she will come up with a different result in one half of her reexaminations, a rather inconsistent performance.

Note immediately that this is not 50% correct—it is 50% reproducible. We do not know the correct results—nor does she. In fact, every result may be incorrect. *Reliability tests are not assessments of correctness.*

Exercise 6.5

□ Suppose now that it really only matters whether the result of the urine examintion is positive (either + or + +) or negative (0). What is the nurse's reliability (or reproducibility) coefficient for this type of labeling?

Comment

First of all, the reproducibility is not necessarily the same as the previous calculation. In fact, the reproducibility is likely to be better than 50% because now the nurse only needs to distinguish between negative and positive (a dichotomous decision), as opposed to distinguishing between 0, +, and + +. Using the data from Table 6.3, Table 6.4 can be constructed.

Table 6.4   **Frequency Distribution of Presence/Absence of Sugar in Urine, by Results of Both Examinations**

		Sugar on exam 1		
		Absent	Present	Total
Sugar on	Absent	10	5	15
exam 2	Present	5	10	15
	Total	15	15	30

Here the reproducibility is (10 + 10)/30 = 67%, which is better than 50%, to be sure, but still not very good.

Exercise 6.6

Urine examination is important as part of the identification of cases of diabetes or their control status in epidemiological studies, as well as in clinical care.

□ Consider the implications of the nurse's reliability for a study of diabetics in which she is involved. (Let us consider her reproducibility for the 0, +, and + + decisions.) Also, consider the implications of her degree of reproducibility for the care of diabetics, if the urine test is used as a guide in their treatment. However, in this context, whether she was correct or not, that is, her accuracy, may be more important than her reproducibility.

Comment

The unreliability of this nurse observer would have consequences in both treatment and epidemiological data-gathering situations. Any inconsistency is damaging in the clinical situation, where the results of such tests may influence clinical judgments and affect a patient's treatment. However, good clinicians often check information from sources known to be unreliable, or they ensure use of reliable sources.

When such information is gathered to indicate the status of groups of individuals (in the form of rates), the consequences may be less hazardous from the individual's point of view, but the resulting data may be useless in reflecting the comparative states of the groups— the data only reflect the observer's acumen (or lack of it) at that moment in time. Some unreliability in studies is to be expected, but if the population or sample is large, a *few* "misses" cannot unduly exaggerate or depress the rates, even if the inconsistency is only in one particular group being compared. However, a few misses can be important if the sample size is much smaller. If reliability is poor, as with the nurse, there will be a lot of uncertainty in defining cases. Any consistent direction of the unreliability can produce false rates; for example, if unreliability on urine specimens is greater in female diabetics than in male diabetics, it will distort the effect measures and the conclusions to be drawn from them.

Exercise 6.7

□ You will recall that this nurse examined the *same* specimens twice. Why did we not have her gather new specimens from the same subjects for her second examination?

Comment

If her second exams had been done on new specimens, even if from the *same subjects*, the test of reproducibility would have been confounded by the biological variability expected to occur between urine samples from the same subject. The natural variability of any characteristic (for example, sugar in urine) over time often presents a problem in checking intra- and interobserver reliability. This is especially true for those characteristics which cannot be gathered and held for future observation (as many laboratory specimens *can* be) or for those which show a high degree of variability within short periods of time (such as blood pressure, pulse rate, emotions).

Exercise 6.8

When more than one person is involved in gathering the data, we are concerned with interobserver reliability; this is measured by the amount of agreement between observers when they measure identical subjects or evidence.

In an actual study in which two physician observers were used to determine cases, an investigation of their reproducibility was carried out. In this investigation, 183 persons were examined independently by both observers and rated as "normal," "Grade 1 byssinosis," or "Grade 2 byssinosis." (Byssinosis, a chronic lung disorder due to inhalation of cotton fibers, is an occupational hazard of textile workers.) The results were as shown in Table 6.5.

Table 6.5   ***Frequency Distribution of Byssinosis Ratings, by Results of Observers A and B, 183 Male Cotton Workers, Aged 40–59***

		Observer A			
		Normal	Grade 1	Grade 2	Total
	Normal	72	6	0	78
	Grade 1	6	47	17	70
Observer B	Grade 2	1	14	20	35
	Total	79	67	37	183

Source: Morris JN: *Uses of Epidemiology, ed 3. Edinburgh and London, E & S Livington, 1975, pp 195–197.*

☐ Calculate the interobserver reliability for the three-way classification, and also for presence (Grades 1 and 2) or absence (normal) of byssinosis.

Comment

The interobserver complete reliability for the three-way classification is (72 + 47 + 20) / 183 = 139/183 or 76%. Reliability on the presence (Grades 1 and 2) or absence (normal) of byssinosis is (72 + 47 + 14 + 17 + 20) /183 = 170/183 = 93%. (There were 14 workers whom observer A rated as Grade 1 and observer B rated as Grade 2.

Similarly, 17 workers were rated as Grade 1 by observer B but Grade 2 by observer A).

The researchers also established the proportion of nonreproducibility between observers A and B on many aspects of diagnosis of the clinical signs of byssinosis, such as chest expansion measurements and gradings of the effect of weather on subjects' breathing.

On that basis, they wrote "observer error is of considerable importance in epidemiological studies when patients are seen once and many of them are normal or have only early manifestations of disease. Much depends on the reliability of single observation of signs and symptoms which are sometimes indefinite.[54]"

Sometimes you will find reliability reported in the form of a correlation coefficient rather than a proportion. A correlation coefficient is a statistical index showing the degree to which one variable changes as another variable changes.

When correlation coefficients are used to measure degrees of reliability, they will range in value from 0 (poor reliability) to 1 (superb reliability). What is "acceptable reliability" depends upon the researcher and the situation, so no hard and fast rule can be given for acceptable values of reliability when a correlation coefficient (or a proportion, for that matter) is used.

Exercise 6.9

□ a. What is the importance of reproducibility in epidemiology?

□ b. What are the sources of nonreproducibility? (Just think logically and about life's examples.)

☐ c. What can be done about these sources of nonreproducibility?

☐ d. From your own experience or knowledge, can you think of health or other characteristics that are "more reliably" and "less reliably" categorized?

Comment

a. Since "to err is human" we never expect or demand complete reproducibility before embarking upon or accepting the findings of an epidemiological investigation. The two examples of reproducibility in this exercise were chosen to illustrate two important aspects of reproducibility. The urine sugar example showed that one observer may be so inconsistent that the findings are little more than an indication of the observer's inconsistency, rather than a true measure of a group's health state.

The byssinosis example showed that when more than one observer is involved, reproducibility *can* reach a high order on "yes or no" criteria, in that case, the presence or absence of byssinosis. It is always more desirable if the errors of observation are randomly dispersed throughout the populations (or samples) surveyed rather than being concentrated in one or the other of the populations (or samples).

As another example of erroneous conclusions that might result from nonrandom systematic mislabeling by more than one observer, consider this illustration. A and B are observers studying disease distribution among men and women. If A examines only men and B examines only women, then nonreproducibility is a potential hazard in comparing the two sexes. That is, differences between the sex-specific disease rates could be due only to the tendency of A and B to differently label certain symptoms in each sex group, rather than due to "real" disease differences between the male and female populations. But if both A and B examine some men and some women and the subjects are randomly assigned to either A or B, then, it is hoped, any errors of A or B are spread throughout the two sex groups. Having A and B both examine men and women helps avoid spurious results obtained by a (potentially) high degree of nonreproducibility (low reliability) of a nonrandom nature.

The important point to remember is that in epidemiological studies, we are seeking information on group differences by characteristics or by disease. Any differences that are produced artificially by labeling tendencies cloud the issue, give false answers to our questions, and must be perpetually guarded against by checks built into the study design.

In every study, therefore, as part of the pretest or planning, an assessment of the intra- and/or interobserver reliability should be obtained, and its dimensions assessed. At least then we will know our errors, correct them, and also be able to consider them as possible explanations of our findings.

b. There are several sources of nonreproducibility, only some of which are attributable to the human observer.

> 1. Sources that are due to the *observer* include: inexperience, carelessness, poor sensory faculties needed to obtain information, previous knowledge or beliefs, variations in methods of applying tests, coding errors, and human biases.

> 2. *Instruments* provide sources, such as leaking mercury from sphygmomanometers (for measuring blood pressure), unreliable measuring scales, and faulty laboratory equipment.

> 3. Sources in the *variable* being measured include: natural biological variability such as blood pressure and pulse rates and subjective phenomena such as anger or happiness.

c. Practice and training of observers reduce unreliability, as does frequent checking and immediate repair (calibration) of any mechanical apparatus. Techniques used in data gathering should be as standardized as possible with a minimum of individual observer difference in method and style.

d. Many clinical tests are not as reliable as we would like them to be; for example, readings of X rays and laboratory tests vary from observer to observer and even from test to test with one observer. All characteristics that vary because of subjective perception on the part of observer or subject run the risk of low reliability. Some examples are emotions, taste, smell, color, or attitude.

Characteristics that are more stable, such as age, sex, or marital status, will have higher reliability; if one sex consistently under-reports age, this will provide high reproducibility even if the information is 100% invalid (incorrect).

Exercise 6.10

Another important piece of the information bias picture is **validity**—the correctness of labeling, the ability of a criterion or tool to measure what it claims to measure, or the correctness of participants' reports.

☐ a. How is validity different from reproducibility?

☐ b. Logically, in terms of validity, in which ways can the presence or the absence of a characteristic be identified correctly or incorrectly?

Comment

a. Validity refers to *correct* measurement or labeling. Theoretically, observers could be 100% reproducible but 100% incorrect (or invalid). That is, they could be very consistant in *mis*labeling, as in our earlier example of consistent underreporting of age by one sex.

b. Quite logically thinking, there are four possibilities. Two ways have to do with how we label people who actually have the diagnosis or characteristic; for convenience we'll refer to these people as cases. The other two possible ways of labeling concern the noncases, those persons who are not positive for the diagnosis or do not have the characteristic.

> 1. We can correctly categorize true cases as cases. We call these **true positives;** this is valid labeling. (It is like calling a spade a spade.)

> 2. We can incorrectly label true cases as noncases. We call these **false negatives.** Obviously such labeling is incorrect or not valid. (It is like calling a spade a pitchfork.)

> 3. We can correctly label the noncases as noncases. These are **true negatives** and the categorization is valid. (It is like correctly calling a pitchfork a pitchfork.)

> 4. We can incorrectly label the noncases as cases. These are **false positives;** obviously this labeling is not valid. (And to complete the alternatives for our simple example, it is like calling a pitchfork a spade.)

Exercise 6.11

Let us return to the example of "urine sugar" to illustrate validity. We ask a technician to test 100 specimens of urine, of which 50 are known to us to contain sugar; the remaining 50 are sugar free.

In the 100 specimens, the technician labeled 65 with sugar, 45 of which were known by us to contain sugar.

☐ a. Complete a frequency distribution table to compare the technician's findings with the known correct results.

☐ b. Calculate the technician's sensitivity and specificity scores. **Sensitivity** is the percentage of all true cases correctly identified—in this instance, a case is sugary urine. **Specificity** is the percentage of all true noncases (with no sugary urine) correctly identified.

Comment

a. Your validity table should resemble Table 6.6.

Table 6.6   **Frequency Distribution of Technician's Test Results, by Actual Absence/Presence of Sugar in 100 Urine Specimens**

		Actual sugar status		
		Present	Absent	Total
Technician's measure of sugar status	Present	(TP) 45	(FP) 20	65
	Absent	(FN) 5	(TN) 30	35
	Total	(Tot P) 50	(Tot N) 50	100

TP = True positive   FN = False negative   Tot P = Total positive
FP = False positive   TN = True negative   Tot N = Total negative

Did constructing this table present difficulties for you? There are enough figures in Exercise 6.11 to do it with some subtraction and addition. It is worth remembering that you do not need the data for *all* the cells in order to construct tables.

b. The technician identified 45 of the 50 true cases (sugary urines) as cases. Therefore, his sensitivity is 45/50 = 90%. He correctly identified 30 of the 50 specimens with no sugar (noncases); therefore, his specificity is 30/50 = 60%.

Sensitivity measures an observer's ability to identify true positives, and specificity identifies an observer's ability to pick out the true negatives. Some prefer to remember *sensitivity* and *specificity* by formulae.

$$\text{Sensitivity} = \frac{\text{TP}}{\text{TP} + \text{FN}} \quad \text{or} \quad \frac{\text{TP}}{\text{TOTAL POS}}$$

$$\text{Specificity} = \frac{\text{TN}}{\text{TN} + \text{FP}} \quad \text{or} \quad \frac{\text{TN}}{\text{TOTAL NEG}}$$

One easy way is to recall that "we should be *sensitive* to cases"; then the rest falls into place. If you need a system for remembering which is which, invent your own.

Exercise 6.12

☐ a. If the technician in Exercise 6.11 works in a screening program to identify individuals for clinical workup, what are the implications of his validity scores (sensitivity and specificity) for the health services system?

☐ b. What is the relevance of validity for epidemiological studies?

Comment

a. His sensitivity rate (90%) indicates that he will not miss identifying many true cases, but his low specificity (60%) suggests that he will mislabel as positive a large number of true negatives and thereby cause an overestimate of cases. This can load a health service with false positives if his test is the basis for patient referral. In addition, it is likely to create unnecessary patient alarm and possibly consequent needless treatment.

For those conditions for which adequate treatment exists and is available, false negatives are especially undesirable, as some cases will not be identified or treated.

b. When information is gathered for descriptive or analytic studies of cause of disease, rather than for service needs, the implications of validity for the individual subject are not as critical. However, incorrectly labeled cases or characteristics may well produce false etiologic associations or mask true causal findings.

Unlike reliability, a determination of validity demands an objective standard of "truth" against which to judge. We may set up as the truth a physician's diagnosis or perhaps standards of growth or biochemical levels. However, as knowledge increases, such standards may change or the decision based upon the standard may change. For many characteristics, standards are not well agreed upon among researchers. There are also some characteristics for which many researchers would say that no standards exist, in which event arbitrary standards are usually established.

Exercise 6.13

☐ a. For some characteristics, the determination of validity may be difficult when an objective standard or set of criteria is not available. Consider health and related characteristics that you feel may be of this sort.

☐ b. What can be done to determine or improve the validity of the measurement of these characteristics?

Comment

a. It is difficult to find a standard for anything that is categorized on the basis of subjective or perceptive assessment. In addition to emotions and sensations of color, smell, or pain, the diagnosis of neurosis and other psychiatric disorders can be very subjective.

b. Unfortunately, often there is little that can be done. Behavioral scientists deal with many variables of this type. In their literature, in addition to "concurrent validity," which is similar to what we have been discussing as validity, you will find such terms as "construct validity" (the measure correlates with the characteristics one would expect it to, so it is probably valid); "face validity" (the measure appears so logical that we accept it at face value as valid); and "predictive validity" (the measure successfully forecasts the outcome of interest).

Predictive validity in epidemiology simply asks the following: Out of the subjects that are labeled as cases, what percentage of them *really are cases?* Obviously, this is an important concept in screening programs. Epidemiologists often utilize the skills and insights of behavioral scientists to better understand modern causes of ill health, so they do come in contact with these other descriptions of validity. But in introductory epidemiological parlance, validity usually refers to sensitivity and specificity.

Exercise 6.14

The data in Table 6.7 are the hypothetical results of two doctors' diagnoses of 30 cases and the correct diagnosis on those cases—correctness being based upon the decision of the "best" clinicians in the world.

Table 6.7   ***Diagnosis, by Physician, and Correct Diagnosis***
                   for 30 Cases

(Hypothetical)

Case number	Dr. A's diagnosis	Dr. B's diagnosis	Correct diagnosis
1	Flu	CHD	Cancer
2	CHD	CHD	CHD
3	Suicide	CHD	CHD
4	Accident	Syphilis	Cancer
5	CHD	CHD	CHD
6	Homicide	Pneumonia	Cancer
7	Stroke	CHD	Flu
8	CHD	Flu	CHD
9	Cancer	CHD	Syphilis
10	CHD	CHD	CHD
11	CHD	CHD	Old age
12	Cancer	CHD	CHD
13	Stroke	CHD	CHD
14	Homicide	Dysentery	Stroke
15	Old age	CHD	Hysteria
16	CHD	CHD	CHD
17	CHD	CHD	CHD
18	Stroke	CHD	CHD
19	CHD	Sclerosis	Accident
20	Accident	Senility	Suicide
21	CHD	CHD	CHD
22	Cancer	Flu	Homicide
23	Drowning	CHD	Cancer
24	Stroke	CHD	CHD
25	Syphilis	Pneumonia	Accident
26	Pneumonia	CHD	CHD
27	Flu	CHD	CHD
28	CHD	CHD	Cancer
29	Pneumonia	CHD	CHD
30	CHD	Syphilis	Psychosis

☐ a. Calculate the interobserver reproducibility of diagnoses
between A and B.

□ b. Calculate the validity (sensitivity and specificity) of Dr. A and of Dr. B for their diagnoses of CHD, using the correct diagnosis as the standard (the truth).

□ c. If one of these two clinicians is to be employed as an examiner for CHD in a screening program prior to full clinical workup, whom would you recommend, A or B? Why?

Comment

a. 8/30 = 26.7%, which suggests that similar training does not ensure high reproducibility. Note that the agreements were all on CHD. On other disorders only, their reproducibility is 0%. If you consider categories of "CHD" or "no CHD" only, they agree 14/30, as shown in Table 6.8.

Table 6.8   *Frequency Distribution of Presence/Absence of CHD, by Physician Observer, for 30 Cases*

		CHD status by Dr. A		
		CHD	No CHD	Total
CHD status by Dr. B	CHD	8	13	21
	No CHD	3	6	9
	Total	11	19	30

On "presence" or "absence" of CHD, they agree 14/30 = 46.7%, as compared with 26.7% reproducibility on all separate diagnoses. In either case, the reliability between these two observers is poor. If both are to be used in a study, we had better train one or both of them and iron out their clinical disparities.

b. Table 6.9 shows the validity of the two diagnoses of the two physicians.

Table 6.9   *Frequency Distribution of Presence/Absence of CHD, by Physician Observer and by Correct Diagnosis for 30 Cases*

		True cases (CHD)	True non-cases (not CHD)	Total
CHD status by Dr. A	CHD	7	4	11
	Not CHD	8	11	19
	Total	15	15	30
CHD status by Dr. B	CHD	14	7	21
	Not CHD	1	8	9
	Total	15	15	30

		Dr. A	Dr. B
Sensitivity $=$	$\dfrac{\text{True positives}}{\text{All true cases}}$	$\dfrac{7}{15} = 46.7\%$	$\dfrac{14}{15} = 93.3\%$
Specificity $=$	$\dfrac{\text{True negatives}}{\text{All noncases}}$	$\dfrac{11}{15} = 73.3\%$	$\dfrac{8}{15} = 53.3\%$

c. Dr. A probably will miss more than half the cases of CHD and is only fairly accurate in identifying noncases. Dr. B has a better record for identifying cases and thus would be the choice for a case-finding and treatment program—that is, if one has the finances and courage to deal with the discontent of a large proportion (46.7%) of people who are incorrectly called cases by Dr. B and the complaints of the follow-up cardiologists.

Exercise 6.15

☐ a. What factors cause variation in the degree of validity?

☐ b. If you find a questionnaire that has been validated by other investigators, can you plan to use it with confidence in your study? Why?

Comment

a. The same types of factors that cause *unreliable* labeling also produce invalid or incorrect labeling, that is, observer characteristics such as inexperience, poor sensory faculties, and previous knowledge and beliefs, as well as instrument sources such as faulty equipment.

In addition, it is obvious that validity is influenced by the choice of the particular standard. Judgments about the best available standard change as knowledge and techniques of diagnosis advance. Thus, it is important in any study to reconsider the validity of all measurement techniques even though they may have been shown valid in the past. In practice, though, many researchers neglect this, a deficiency that may haunt them when they interpret their findings.

b. Not necessarily. Some studies have shown that validity is not constant across all groups; the validity of the same test instrument can be different among different ethnic groups, for example. This has important implications, for it suggests that the degree of validity determined previously for a particular group of subjects may not hold true for the groups you wish to study or even for a similar group at another point in time. It is worth reestablishing the validity in each subpopulation if some degree of confidence in the results is to be enjoyed.

In addition to the possible need to establish cross-cultural validity for your own study, the assumption that your study staff is validly labeling variables must also be investigated.

Summary

The main points covered in this chapter include:

1. Information bias or incorrect labeling of cases, characteristics, or other variables consists of two components: reproducibility and validity.

2. Reproducibility (reliability or repeatability) is assessed as the degree of agreement between two or more observers (interobserver) or within one observer (intra-observer) on repeat tests.

3. Reliability varies with the skills of the observer, the variability of the characteristic being measured, and the consistency of instruments used.

4. Reliability can be improved by training of observers and calibration of instruments or tests.

5. Validity is an indication of the correctness of labeling. It comprises sensitivity (percentage of true cases identified) and specificity (percentage of true noncases identified).

6. Both validity and reliability have implications for research and health services activities.

References and Further Reading Sources

Topic	Reference number	Pages
Reliability (reproducibility or repeatability)	1	85–94
	40	248
	42	(article)
	45	195–196
	54	(article)
	68	30–36
Validity	1	95–105
	2	(article)
	22	(article)
	24	214–226
	34	456–476
	38	261–265
	40	424–252
	45	42–44
	68	36–49

Method Pitfall 2:
Potential Hazards in Classifying Data

7

In the previous chapter, we considered whether observations or measurements made were reliable and valid, as well as implications of unreliability and nonvalidity.

In this chapter, we consider the classification of observations and its potential hazards. In epidemiology we often classify persons into groups or categories such as diseased or not diseased, upper or lower social class, and it is necessary to define criteria for each group. The criteria will depend upon current knowledge of the health outcome or other characteristics and upon the type of data we have available—whether the data are quantitative, such as blood pressure, or categorical, such as marital or pregnancy status or sex. In classification, we may lose useful information and mask conclusions.

All too often we make arbitrary decisions in these classifications, but that is fine as long as we understand the compromises we accept in so doing.

Exercise 7.1

Table 7.1 shows some hypothetical blood pressure recordings on 20 persons.

☐ a. Can you tell from the data in the table whether the measurement of systolic and diastolic blood pressure is reliable? How?

Write down your answer, then read the following discussion.

**Table 7.1   Systolic and Diastolic Blood Pressure (BP)
reading on 20 Persons**

Person	Systolic BP (in mm Hg)	Diastolic BP (in mm Hg)	Person	Systolic BP (in mm Hg)	Diastolic BP (in mm Hg)
1	160	90	11	120	80
2	212	74	12	164	92
3	110	54	13	156	92
4	162	86	14	200	88
5	146	94	15	120	64
6	184	64	16	150	96
7	200	110	17	148	84
8	158	94	18	210	110
9	140	60	19	140	86
10	210	86	20	160	88

☐ b. Can you tell from the data in the table whether the measurement is valid? How?

Comment

a. No. No information is given about who measured the blood pressure or whether one or more observers was used. And even then, this table gives no indication of interobserver or intra-observer reliability.

b. No. There are no validity data in this table.

Exercise 7.2

What is the rate of hypertension (high BP) among the 20 subjects in Table 7.1 if one categorizes a subject as hypertensive when BP is:

□ a. Systolic = 160 mm or more?

□ b. Diastolic = 90 mm or more?

□ c. Systolic = 160 mm or more or diastolic = 90 mm or more?

□ d. Systolic = 160 mm or more *and* diastolic = 90 mm or more?

Comment

a. With this cutoff point, the rate of hypertension is 10/20 = 50%.

b. This rate would be 8/20 = 40%.

c. This rate would be 14/20 = 70%.

You should avoid merely adding (a) and (b) to get (c), for some patients fit into both (a) and (b), but get counted only once in (c). It is correct to count each hypertensive case only once.

d. Under these cutoff points, a subject labeled as hypertensive must have *both* high systolic and diastolic readings to be counted in the numerator, which would make the rate 4/20 = 20%.

Exercise 7.3

☐ What are the implications of your answers for comparing different studies of hypertension?

Comment

As you see, the rates of hypertension in this small sample of 20 subjects change from 20% to 70% as we vary the classification criteria. The rates can be further changed by choosing different blood pressure levels as the cutoff points to define hypertension.

Thus, studies that use different criteria for defining presence of any health state are not comparable with respect to reported rates of that health state. The use of different criteria or definitions in classification is a problem that can be solved only by cooperative decision by researchers. For example, epidemiological committees have urged general usage of agreed-upon cutoff points for blood pressure. Because of this, hypertension studies using these criteria can be compared to each other with more confidence.

This is not to imply, however, that epidemiological results are strictly comparable if identical diagnostic criteria were used. The investigations may differ on any of the other important methodological points that we consider.

All study reports you or others make should clearly state the criteria used for classifying variables. When deciding upon classification criteria for your own investigations, there is value in using criteria of other researchers even if it means reporting your results in more than one way—one way using the criteria that *you* see as conceptually most desirable and another way for comparability purposes.

Exercise 7.4

□ a. Is blood pressure a quantitative or categorical variable?

□ b. Is hypertension a quantitative or categorical variable?

□ c. What results from categorizing quantitative data?

Comment

a. BP is a quantitative variable; the number for BP indicates the amount of pressure.

b. Hypertension is a categorical variable (also called "nominal," from a Latin word that means "name"). In this example, subjects are either hypertensive or not. The quantitative blood pressure measurement has been used to create two categories based on the concept that high blood pressure (hypertension) is a disease entity.

c. Loss of useful information may result.

Some information on variability between persons is lost when quantitative data are categorized. For example, all those persons classified as hypertensive by having systolic BP of 160 or more are now regarded as identical to each other even though these persons do not have identical BP measurements.

Collapsing a quantitative variable into a categorical variable with two or more categories may also obscure the fact that the underlying variable has a much larger range in one category than in another category. (Note: the *range* of a collection of observations is the largest observation minus the smallest observation.) For example, at the cutoff point of 90 mm or more diastolic BP in this example, the range for hypertensives is 20 (90 to 110) whereas the range for nonhypertensives is 34 (54 to 88). Be careful, though, about comparing ranges in general because a larger sample will generally have a larger range. Here, one reason that the range may be larger in the nonhypertensive group is that there are 12 subjects in that group compared with only 8 in the hypertensive group.

Collapsing quantitative variables into categories also limits the choices of appropriate statistical tests of significance you may want to use.

However, there are positive results from categorization. Without it, we would never be able to calculate rates for some health states and compare them. Further, some categories have ecological meaning or social meaning. For example, we often use age 65 as "old" because so many legislative, health, and other services use this cutoff point. Further commonly used categories such as five- or ten-year age bands in available data, for example, from census, encourage our use of those same categories.

On occasion, the biological meaning of a cutoff point on a quantitative variable is confirmed, thereby providing support for clinical intervention. These categorical cutoff points, however, are frequently debated and do change as knowledge advances.

Exercise 7.5

☐ Applying these considerations, what thoughts do you have in using age as a variable?

Comment

Often, as pertaining to adults, one uses five-year age bands, such as 20–24 and 25–29. But in studying infants, we know now that they are very different in respect to death, causes of death, and diseases in the first few days of life, as compared with the first four weeks and later weeks. Thus, we often categorize ages in infancy as perinatal (first week of life), neonatal (first 28 days of life) and postneonatal, or 29 days to one year. So our knowledge, our conceptual question, and other published information must guide us.

In general, it is advisable not to start with wide ranges of categories, such as 20-year age bands, but rather with smaller components of the large category, such as five-year age bands. If adjacent smaller categories do not differ on the health state, and are not important in the test of the hypothesis or for other purposes, then you may wish to combine them into a larger category since you are not masking any differences in doing so.

Exercise 7.6

Table 7.2   **Classification of 100 Consecutive Patients in an Out-patient Clinic**

Category	Patients
Bacterial infection	40
Anxiety	53
Cancer	10
Localized infection	15
Old age	8
Tiredness	3

☐ a. Is the classification in Table 7.2 useful at all?

□ b. Can you modify it to be more useful for epidemiological purposes?

□ c. What characterizes classification systems in epidemiology?

Comment

a. Yes, but it depends upon the use to which it is to be put.
This might be a useful classification scheme for specialists within the
clinic. The psychiatrist may want to know how many people have anxiety, no matter what additional afflictions they might have.

b. Some patients have double (or more) pathology and so
appear in more than one category; this is obvious because the sum of
the diagnostic frequencies (patients columns) is greater than 100. This
problem of nonexclusive categories can be solved by creating separate
categories or combinations of disorders such as anxiety *and* cancer. Or
persons with double or triple pathology, along with the patients with
pathologies not mentioned in the list, could be put in a category called
"other," but this "catch-all" category is not very helpful, and may be
detrimental if it includes many people.

Remember that **mutually exclusive categories** only allow a
subject to appear in one of those categories. **Exhaustive categories** are
such that all subjects are classifiable and can appear once in *some*

category (as provided for by the "other" category in the example). The category of "other" may become necessary when all possible expected categories are not known; it is often included just in case some unanticipated entity turns up.

c. All persons in the study must be classifiable. Clearly this may require some additional categories such as "refused to answer," "missing data," "unknown," and "other."

Criteria for each classification should be laid down and strictly applied. The classification system must have meaning conceptually as related to the study purpose.

Summary

The main points covered in Chapter 7 include:

1. Choice of categories for quantitative variables can affect the results.

2. Loss of information and analytical power in our statistical tests may follow such categorization.

3. For comparability with other studies, arbitrary cutoff points are sometimes recommended for classification purposes and used in many studies.

4. In determining categories, the use of smaller ranges initially is indicated. Categories with large ranges may mask important differences if decided upon before examination of the data.

5. Classificatory systems should permit all persons in the study to be classified, and only once, including "refusal, unknown, missing data" categories; that is, they should be exhaustive and exclusive.

6. These characteristics should be considered at the commencement of a study when variables and classificatory schemes are being considered for use in the study.

References and Further Reading Sources

Topic	Reference number	Pages
Variables and their classification	1	46–64
	24	353–368
	38	47–55
	40	5–9

Method Pitfall 3:
Selection Bias—Who Gets In?

8

In the previous two chapters, we learned about the potential pitfalls associated with information bias—the error in the incorrect labeling of cases and noncases and problems associated with categorization of data. Another set of considerations confronts us in regard to the sorts of populations we study and their relevance to how we interpret data and what inferences we can draw.

This chapter is concerned with who gets into an epidemiological study—as participants, not as investigators. It addresses the population at risk and the forces of **selection** that can produce incorrect findings, in the sense that the findings are not based upon the correct populations. This selection bias (which refers to the distortion of effect measures resulting from the way participants get into studies) is an important "pitfall," an area of potential error.

Exercise 8.1

In a hypothetical study, the prevalence rate of transplanted heart patients was higher in Stanford, California in 1980 than in any other city of the world.

☐ Why would this be a likely finding?

Write down your answer, then read the following discussion.

Comment

The Stanford University surgical expertise attracts those in need of this service. This is a very simple example of the effect of *selective use of health services* in producing a finding. Obviously we would be drawing a false conclusion if we decided that something about Stanford other than the surgeons' presence was associated with the high rate of transplanted hearts in Stanford.

Another classic example of this type of selection was the initial description of the occurrence of thromboangeitis obliterans (Buerger's disease—a disease affecting the peripheral blood vessels). In 1908 when Leo Buerger originally described the syndrome, he wrote, "The disease occurs frequently, although not exclusively, among the Polish and Russian Jews and it is in the dispensaries and hospitals of New York City that we find a good opportunity for studying it. . . ." (*Am J Med Sci* 136: 567, 1908)

It now seems likely that *any* disorder then described by Buerger would have appeared to be more common among Polish and Russian Jews for he worked at Mt. Sinai Hospital in New York, which at that time was used almost exclusively by Jews of Polish and Russian extraction.

So the sort of clientele (the characteristics of the population) using a health service may well determine an association that is not really epidemiologically significant. Such an association is artifactual and hence "noncausal," produced as it was by selection bias.

Exercise 8.2

Hollingshead and Redlich studied psychiatric cases diagnosed and reported by psychiatrists and mental health agencies in a community. The associations they found between mental illness and social class are shown in Table 8.1

Table 8.1   ***Prevalence Rates* per 100,000 of Psychosis and Neurosis by Social Class Categories (Sex- and Age-Adjusted), Connecticut, 1950***

	Social class	Psychosis	Neurosis
High	1 & 2	188	349
	3	291	250
	4	518	114
Low	5	1,505	97

*These rates were based upon people diagnosed by these practitioners. The data do not come from a population survey.

Source: Hollingshead AB, Redlich FC: *Social Class and Mental Illness.* New York, John Wiley & Sons, 1958, p. 235.

☐ a. Was this a cohort, case-control, or cross-sectional study?

☐ b. From Table 8.1, what is the association of social class with psychosis and with neurosis?

Comment

a. If you have become accustomed to reading table headings, you will realize that prevalence rates are derived from cross-sectional (point prevalence) studies. Remember to read titles of tables.

Note also that rates are sex and age adjusted. From previous exercises, we understand age adjustment, but sex adjustment? It does not sound logical or desirable, but just recall from Chapter 1 that nothing changes actually in adjustment. This is merely a statistical manipulation to prevent drawing erroneous conclusions due to unequal distribution of sexes among the social classes. Also, remember that the adjustment is needed only if mental illness and the characteristic of sex are associated (they are associated, in fact). In any case, if sexes are equally distributed in the classes, then no adjustment on sex is necessary either.

b. There appears to be an inverse or negative association between social class and psychosis (the higher the social class, the lower the psychosis rate), and a direct or positive association between social class and neurosis (the higher the social class, the higher the neurosis rate). The associations were tested to be statistically significant.

Exercise 8.3

Before accepting these associations at face value, we must consider alternative explanations to a "real" relationship or association.

☐ a. Could factors of information bias produce these results? If so, how? Recall that this bias refers to false labeling.

☐ b. What factors of selection bias could produce these results? Recall that selection bias relates to the nature of the populations studied.

Comment

a. They certainly could. Here we start thinking of logical possibilities.

Reproducibility

There are few agreed-upon diagnostic criteria for the clinical syndromes of neurosis and psychosis. So intra-observer and inter-observer reliability may be low, which has been shown to be true. Either one of these aspects of reliability can produce artifactual differences in the rates of neuroses and psychoses among the social classes. One observer may apply different criteria for neurosis and psychosis in different social classes, resulting in low intra-observer reliability *and* an artifactual difference in rates among social classes. Similarly, two observers may apply different criteria in different social classes *or* they each may apply their own criteria consistently in all social classes but differ from each other on the criteria. If each observer sees subjects primarily from different social classes, then this low interobserver reliability could produce artificial differences in rates among social classes, as in Table 8.1.

Validity

The people doing the labeling were middle- and upper-class people, such as psychiatrists and practitioners, who may prefer to label their upper-class peers neurotic rather than psychotic as there would be less stigma to neurosis. Also, because neurosis infers better prognosis, treatment would more likely be obtained by the patient. In other words, the degree of validity could differ in the different social classes. That is, the same disorder is called one thing for upper-class people and another thing for those in the lower class. Perhaps because of the diagnosticians' class affiliation (medical practitioners are generally placed in upper social classes), they did not understand the behavior and responses of those in other classes which, in turn, could lead to invalid diagnoses and labeling. This could also cause validity to vary by the class characteristics of subjects. These do not exhaust the possibilities of bias as an alternative explanation, but they illustrate the point. You can think of other ways in which the class of the subject can influence diagnostic labeling.

b. One factor of selection might be that lower-class neurotics do not have the ability, inclination, or money to seek diagnosis or treatment to the extent that upper-class neurotics do. If so, they would not get into the services or treatment net to become labeled and counted (an example of selective use of services). They may come to the diagnosticians' attention only when seriously ill with psychosis.

We must be alert also to possibilities of selection *out* of the epidemiological net. Perhaps psychotic upper-class people choose and are able to leave their geographic area because their behavior is at odds with accepted behavior for their group. If this happens, those who are seriously ill (psychotics) would not be around for labeling in the study (an example of "selective out-migration").

Because this is a cross-sectional or prevalence study, we must be particularly aware that the disease (dependent variable) can place an individual in one or another category of the independent variable. Psychotics may drift down the social ladder because of their illness. Also, there may be something about neurotics that makes them social climbers ("selective interclass migration"). As you will recall in cross-sectional studies, cause and effect considerations are not answerable— either characteristic could "cause" the other.

Thus, information bias and selection bias could produce the results in Table 8.1 and create "noncausal," artifactual associations by distorting the effect measures (the rates).

We always should consider biases as possible explanations of findings before proceeding to other hypothesized processes to explain the associations. We suggest you consider these potential conclusions from your own studies.

Exercise 8.4

The map opposite, adapted from the classical study by Faris and Dunham, depicts the prevalence rates of schizophrenia in Chicago in the 1930s.

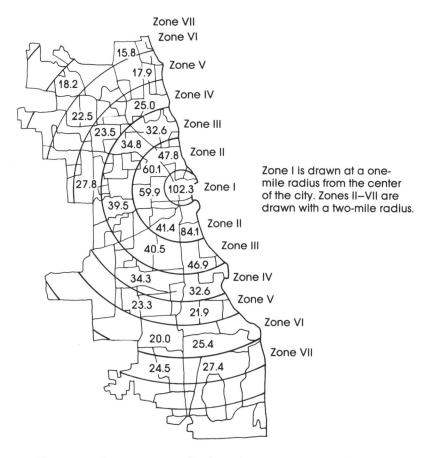

Zone I is drawn at a one-mile radius from the center of the city. Zones II–VII are drawn with a two-mile radius.

Figure 8.1 Average rates of schizophrenia, 1922–1934, by geographic zones and divisions of Chicago.
(Rates per 100,000 population, aged 15–64, 1930.) Subcommunities are based on census tracts of Chicago.

Source: Adapted from Faris R, Dunham HW, *Mental Disorders in Urban Areas.* University of Chicago Press, 1939.

☐ a. Comment upon the patterns of the rates.

☐ b. What forces of selection bias and information bias could produce these findings?

Comment

This map is famous in the annals of the epidemiology of
schizophrenia. Note that rates are not age-adjusted, so we must be alert
as to whether age is a confounding variable producing an artifactual
association.

a. Rates are higher in the center city zone and generally
decrease as the concentric zones radiate outward. There are no great
differences in the rates between the divisions within each zone.

b. As in the previous example, this association may not be
due to where the people were currently situated on the independent
variable (distance from center city in this case).

Perhaps schizophrenics move to the center city for treatment.
Or living in the center city may be easier for schizophrenics than living
in the suburbs, and hence schizophrenics selectively migrate into the
center city. Maybe there is a labeling bias against diagnosing schizophrenia among suburbanites. Or perhaps suburbanites are more for-
tunate in their cure ratio (unlikely, as yet). Again, perhaps suburban
schizophrenics are banished elsewhere (for example, to the center city)
for their cure or because of their socially "unacceptable" behavior. Perhaps there is an added risk factor that causes schizophrenics to die at
a higher rate in the suburbs than in the center city (different case fatality
rates), so fewer cases survive to be counted in this prevalence study.

Because this is a prevalence study, we are merely applying
the possible explanations that you learned in previous exercises—factors such as selective mortality, migration, and different case fatality
or cure ratios.

Exercise 8.5

□ Consider and list the general categories of force of selection that can produce spurious, artifactual results and associations.

Comment

Selective use of services, selective migration in or out of the study area, selective social mobility, selective mortality/survival/cure—all of these may be due to the health state in question, or some antecedent of it, or other characteristics. All of these possibilities must be considered in looking at study findings, especially when they are in terms of prevalence. Sometime at your convenience read Faris and Dunham[23] for a discussion of these possibilities.

Despite these confounding possibilities, many findings go on to become scientific facts, often by other studies replicating findings or by attention in substudies to eliminate these alternate explanations. The findings of Faris and Dunham have stood the test of time and replication.

Exercise 8.6

□ Consider and write down some of the selective forces on study populations that can operate in all epidemiological studies and may produce spurious associations.

Comment

1. Volunteers for studies are almost invariably selective, often in terms of their health attributes. Sometimes they fear that they have (or do not have) the condition you are studying or sometimes they volunteer because they are very healthy.

2. Paid participants may be selectively different from the general population, especially if they are informed about payment before they participate.

3. Hospital and clinic data are invariably based on a selective population. The statistician Joseph Berkson pointed out the fallacy that this produces (called Berkson's fallacy) because associations found from hospital (or clinic) data are influenced by the differential admission rates among groups of people. A similar fallacy is applicable to associations based upon autopsy data.

Some recent controversial issues have been initiated by publication of associations established for hospital patients that later have been refuted when tested in nonhospital populations. An example is the association of reserpine (a drug used for lowering blood pressure) and breast cancer, established in studies in hospitals but subsequently refuted.

4. Studies of illness in industrial working popula-

tions have shown that their risk of certain illnesses is lower than that in the general population. This is probably not due to the health-promotive environment of industries (it may be) but rather to the so-called healthy worker effect, which results from preemployment examinations usually precluding ill people from being employed. This effect may decline with time as any ill health effects of industries create illnesses in initially healthy workers.

Further readings about selective factors are referenced at the end of this chapter.

Summary

The main points covered in Chapter 8 include:

1. Forces of selection can produce biased estimates of the effect.

2. These include selective use of services, selective migration, and selective mortality or survival.

3. They relate to people choosing various services or places, often because of illness, in order to be allowed to stay in an accepting area or to be employed. These forces must be considered in interpreting findings, for they may create associations that cannot be causal.

References and Further Reading Sources

Topic	Reference number	Pages
Selective factors	17	(article)
	23	160–177
	29	25–39
	36	169–176
	45	51–56
Berkson's fallacy	7	(article)
	11	(article)
	39	(article)
	49	(article)

However, reconsidering the data on an individual basis, only 3/6 or 50% of the young people are sick whereas 4/4 or all of the old people are sick. Thus, a larger percentage of old people are ill, which refutes the absence of the typical association of sickness with age found when group indices were compared.

Exercise 9.2

In his classic study of suicide in the late 1800s, Durkheim associated suicide with religion, as shown in Table 9.2.

Table 9.2   *Suicide Rates per Million* by Proportion of Catholics in Bavarian Provinces, 1867–1875*

Provinces with <50% Catholic		Provinces with 50–90% Catholic		Provinces with >90% Catholic	
Province	Rate	Province	Rate	Province	Rate
RP	167	LF	157	UP	64
CF	207	Sa	118	UB	114
UF	204			LB	19
Average	192		135		75

*The population under 15 years old has been omitted.

Source: Durkheim E, Suicide, in Simpson G (ed): *A Study in Sociology,* Glencoe, Ill, The Free Press, 1951. By permission of Macmillan Publishing Co., Inc., and Routledge and Kegan Paul, Ltd.

Durkheim wrote the following about his findings:

On the other hand, if one compares the different provinces of Bavaria, suicides are found to be in direct proportion to the number of Protestants, and in inverse proportion to that of Catholics. Not only the proportions of averages to one and the other confirm the law, but all the numbers of the first column are higher than those of the second, and those of the second higher than those of the third without exception. (21, p 153)

☐ Would you agree that the data in the table support the finding of an inverse association between suicide and Catholicism? Why or why not?

Comment

Durkheim has used two ecologic or group indices and compared them, namely, suicide rate and proportion of Catholics. This is potentially fallacious. Perhaps in provinces with over 90% Catholic, the Protestant minority committed suicide at a high rate and the Catholic majority at a low rate, whereas in provinces with a Catholic minority, the Catholics may have had a high suicide rate and the Protestants a moderate suicide rate. Durkheim's general conclusion or suggestion is that *rates of suicide for all Catholics are low,* which cannot be proven by these data alone.

Exercise 9.3

☐ What could he have done to avoid the problem of an ecologic fallacy?

Comment

He could have calculated, if possible, religion-specific rates of suicide in each province. Each religious group in the province should have its own suicide rate with only its membership in the numerator and denominator. Durkheim actually did precisely that for many countries and presented "directly determined" rates from information about suicide and religion on an individual basis. His treatise on suicide is well worth reading.[21]

Exercise 9.4

□ Note in Table 9.2 that 192 is *not* the average of the three numbers 167, 207, 204. What kind of average is 192?

Comment

The 192 is a **weighted** average of 167, 207, and 204, where the province with the largest population gets the largest weight and the province with the smallest population gets the smallest weight. The weighted average 192 can be interpreted as follows: If the populations of the three provinces RP, CF, and UF were added together and one suicide rate calculated for the combined provinces, the rate would be 192.

To reiterate, just taking the average of the three numbers 167, 207, and 204 would yield an **unweighted** average of the suicide rates, which would not be appropriate *unless* all three provinces were of the same size with respect to population.

Exercise 9.5

□ Certain characteristics are well suited to ecologic (group) indices and tend to be more useful than others. Can you think of any examples?

Comment

If a town has only one water supply, its content of a mineral or chemical such as lead, DDT, or any other is likely to be fairly constant for all inhabitants. So it may be useful to consider several such towns and compare the quantity of lead in each town's water source with the rate of some health characteristic. Although the amount of lead received by persons in a given town is fairly constant, it *does* depend upon the amount of water each person drinks and how much of the intake does *not* come from the town source, be it from imported beer, rainwater, or transatlantic moonshine.

Indices of air pollution in neighborhoods are also good indicators of individual pollution exposure, even with air conditioning. Some individuals may be exposed to additional or different pollution, for example, by virtue of occupation. One just applies logic and common sense in assessing the relative merits of using any ecologic index in a particular situation and confirms the applicability of the ecologic index by testing it, if possible, in a sample of individuals.

Exercise 9.6

In another classic study in 1849, Dr. Snow, in associating cholera with the water source, presented the comparison of mortality shown in Table 9.3.

Table 9.3   **Number of Deaths per 10,000 Houses in Population Supplied by Three Water Companies During Seven-Week Epidemic**

Water supply	Houses	Deaths from cholera	Deaths per 10,000 houses
Southwark and Vauxhall Co	40,046	1,263	315
Lambeth Co	26,107	98	37
Rest of London	256,423	1,422	59

Source: Richardson BW: *Snow on Cholera.* New York: The Commonwealth Fund, 1936, p 186.

□ Is this another example of the potential ecologic fallacy? Why do you think that?

Comment

No. Snow calculated a specific rate for each water source, a rate of cholera deaths per 10,000 houses receiving water from one source only. Later he moved from the less precise rate of deaths per 10,000 houses to the more specific rate of deaths per 10,000 population, which further proved his hypothesis. His book *On the Mode of Communication of Cholera* is an easy-to-read delight. That he was not a professional epidemiologist should encourage you to practice epidemiology whatever your professional bent.

Exercise 9.7

In a more modern study, the association of hardness of water and mortality from coronary heart disease and cerebrovascular disease was examined. In contrast to the generally shown negative asociation of water hardness and CHD deaths, the findings shown in Table 9.4 failed to demonstrate a simple relationship of average water hardness to coronary heart disease mortality.

Table 9.4   *Average Water Hardness and Death Rates of White Men Aged 55–64 From Coronary Heart Disease and Cerebrovascular Disease, Regions of North Carolina, 1956–1964*

Region	Average hardness (in ppm of CaCo$_3$)	Average annual death rate (per 100,000) Coronary heart disease	Average annual death rate (per 100,000) Cerebrovascular disease
Highland	23	585	147
Piedmont	61	778	172
Coastal plain	51	877	247
Tidewater	163	713	218

Source: From Tyroler HA: Epidemiologic studies of cardiovascular disease in three communities of the southeastern United States, in Kessler II, Levin M (eds): *The Community as an Epidemiologic Laboratory: A Casebook of Community Studies*, Baltimore: Johns Hopkins Press, 1970. ©1970 The Johns Hopkins University Press.

☐ Is this an example of the use of ecologic indices? Is this potentially fallacious?

☐ Why do you think so?

Comment

Yes, and *potentially* fallacious. Here the researchers have lumped together counties with different water supplies into a regional average for water hardness and associated that average with mortality from CHD and cerebrovascular disease. Clearly, these indices cannot actually assess whether more men aged 55 to 64 drinking hard water in a county or region died from those diseases than those drinking soft water, assuming that different sources of water (for example, wells) are available in a county. However, these findings merit further study at an individual level because of their potential importance.

Exercise 9.8

☐ What could the investigators have done in the water hardness study to reduce any sort of fallacy?

Comment

They could have measured the hardness of the water supply of each person and then associated that with CHD death rates derived from individual death certificates. Or they could have carried out the investigation in each of the 100 counties of North Carolina where residents may have a more consistently uniform water supply. However, such studies are often difficult, especially in rural areas where water comes from rainwater storages or wells that have not been tested for water hardness.

Exercise 9.9

☐ Because of the potential fallacy, should the use of ecologic indices be avoided? Why?

Comment

No, not entirely. Because of the ready availability of ecologic indices—be they disease rates or demographic, social, agricultural, or environmental indices—they lend themselves fairly easily to generating hypotheses and testing hunches. Some of the greatest epidemiological discoveries were based upon the use of ecologic indices. These include the association of Burkitt's lymphoma with malaria, the sickling trait with malaria mortality, and yellow fever with the mosquito. One can only presume, in assessing these studies, that the association was so strong that any fallacy was overridden or that the assumptions made in using the ecologic indices were correct.

Just remember that ecologic studies, unless they can create specific rates for subpopulations, are not proof of an association. Because ecologic indices can produce incorrect associations or fail to reveal existing ones, use your logic in assessing the extent of the possible error when judging articles that report this technique or when using the technique yourself. Their use can be most productive if accompanied by wariness, thought, and further study. Such considerations should be included in the interpretation of associations found between ecologic (or group-based) indices. Many other studies, especially in the field of environmental epidemiology, use ecologic indices, for example, studies of radiation, air pollution, pesticides, and lead.

Summary

The main points covered in this chapter include:

1. Consideration is given to the potential error (ecologic fallacy) that can arise in associating groups or ecologic indices with health outcomes.

2. Such an ecologic index assumes that the index reflecting a common characteristic in a group is applicable to all members of the group.

3. The fallacy is avoidable by using measurements derived from the individual's characteristics.

4. Ecologic indices are available and most useful in developing ideas for associations or supporting hunches.

5. Logic should be used in assessing the extent of the fallacy.

6. Interpretation of associations between ecologic indices should be reviewed carefully and warily.

References and Further Reading Sources

Topic	Reference number	Pages
Ecologic indices	21	152–170
	23	152–156
	35	100–122
	57	1–98

Cohort Effect: Looking at a
Particular Group Through Time

10

We have already considered group indices and the possible fallacy involved in using such ecologic indices in the interpretation of associations. When data suggest the possibility that they are demonstrating the experience of one *particular group* over time, such a group is referred to as a cohort. Its effect is termed a "cohort effect," borrowed from the use of cohort in ancient Roman days to refer to a group of warriors. You recall we used the same term in describing one of the strategies used in epidemiology, namely, the cohort or prospective method. In this chapter, we are considering a cohort as a particular or unique group that shares some common experience relevant to health.

Exercise 10.1

□ What sort of groups can you think of that would fit this description?

Write down your answer, then read the following discussion.

Comment

Some examples of cohorts are people born in the same year or decade (birth cohorts), cohorts exposed to a war, cohorts exposed to radiation from the atomic bomb explosions of 1945, or persons exposed to a drug that is subsequently taken off the market (such as the daughters of mothers who took diethylstilbesterol during pregnancy). You may think of others.

Exercise 10.2

Figure 10.1 depicts the hypothetical association of a disease with age in 1970. We saw this sort of association in Chapter 2 on cross-sectional strategy. The data are from a cross-sectional design.

□ How can these findings be explained by a birth cohort effect?

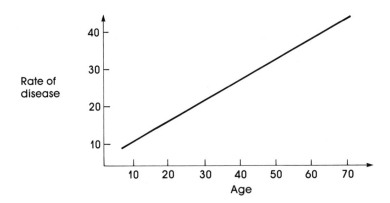

Figure 10.1 Disease prevalence rate per 100,000, by age, 1970 (hypothetical).

Comment

One explanation of an association of any disease with age in the particular year when the cross-sectional study was done is that the particular old people of that year *always* had a higher rate than any other age group through time. That means they had the highest rate when they were 60 years old, when they were 50, 40, or whenever.

Exercise 10.3

If a birth cohort effect is the explanation for the association in Figure 10.1, then the particular old people in 1970 always had higher rates through time.

☐ Which age group would show the highest rate in 1960?

Comment

The rate would be highest in the 60-year-olds. If this unique expression of disease began early in life, then the rate in 1900 would be the highest among infants.

Exercise 10.4

☐ Can you think of a disorder that could show this age cohort effect, that is, be highly prevalent at birth and persist in that birth cohort through time?

Comment

One thinks of a nonfatal persistent birth disorder. An example could be the cohort of "thalidomide babies" in Europe (if they were common enough to be seen in a big population) or a cohort of blind babies exposed to overadministration of oxygen at birth (the retrolental fibroplasia syndrome). The thalidomide babies were born in the early 1960s and the retrolental fibroplasia syndrome occurred around the same period.

Thus, in 1980 in Europe (the United States was spared the widespread use of thalidomide and its consequences) there will be a relatively high rate of thalidomide-affected adults among those aged 20, compared with others younger or older.

Another similar nondisease birth cohort recognized by demographers is the baby-boom babies of the late 1940s. (The baby boom refers to the high rate that followed the Second World War.) This birth cohort created a great need for college places in the 1960s and 1970s, a need that would disappear in the early 1980s, giving education administrators cause for concern.

Exercise 10.5

☐ Can you think of other age cohorts manifesting a high rate of a disorder in a particular period of time, which then persists with them into older age?

Comment

Veterans of war who were disabled, such as draftees aged 18 to 19 in 1970–1973 who were crippled by the Vietnam War. If no war breaks out in the interim, they will show a higher rate of amputations, crippling, and so forth at age 30 to 31 in the 1982–1985 as compared with people younger and up to 25 or less years older than themselves. Similarly, we are now still aware of a high rate of leukemia and radiation effects in people who were exposed to the atomic bombs in Hiroshima and Nagasaki in 1945. Those afflicted are now older, manifesting higher rates of radiation-related disease than persons born later or earlier. Continuing with this thought process, mothers who were exposed to the bomb's radiation while pregnant may produce a birth cohort of defective babies.

Exercise 10.6

Figure 10.2 gives the distribution of the prevalence of dental caries among Black men in North Carolina in 1960–1963, as measured by the DMF Index (decayed, missing, and filled teeth). We all know

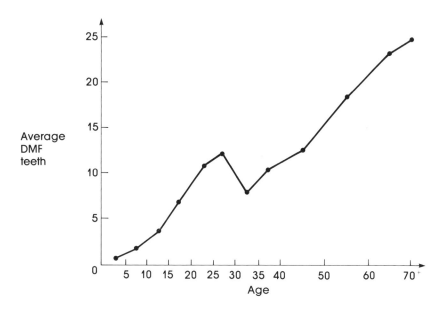

Figure 10.2 Average DMF for Black men, by age, North Carolina, 1960–1963.

Source: Fulton JT and Hughes JT: *The Natural History of Dental Diseases.* Chapel Hill, Department of Epidemiology, University of North Carolina, 1965.

that dental caries never get better as age increases, nor are they fatal. One's aching tooth gets "pulled, plugged, or putrid," any of which labels that tooth as DMF forever. An edentulous (toothless) person would have a DMF of 32; an adult with all 32 teeth filled would get the same score.

☐ a. Describe the shape of the distribution of average DMF in Figure 10.2.

☐ b. If any suggeston of a cohort phenomenon exists, what additional steps would you take now to confirm it?

Comment

a. This is a bimodal distribution with two peaks (modes), at ages 25 to 29 and 70+, and dips at ages 30 to 34 and 35 to 39. In this instance of dental caries, this is very suggestive of a cohort effect among those 30 to 39 years old in 1960. This age cohort has an unusually *low* rate, lower than older persons but also lower than younger persons.

A note on bimodality: one sees multiple modes in distributions of disease prevalence or death rates in a fair number of conditions, for example, leukemia has a peak (mode) in 2- to 5-year-olds and then a later peak in persons over 55. This suggests either two separate populations or diseases or else a cohort effect. Thus, with leukemia, the young people may have a different disorder from those with the disease in older age. This has been confirmed clinically, for the disease is usually an acute type in youth and a more chronic type in older people. This also suggests different causation networks for each syndrome.

Similar suggestive evidence of two different syndromes and two different causations is seen in diabetes prevalence by age, deaths from automobile accidents by age, and Down's syndrome by mother's age.

    b. First, it would seem reasonable to see if this cohort effect is reflected in other sex-ethnic groups. In fact, it was found in men and women among both Blacks and Whites. Then, this cohort effect could be confirmed by repeating the prevalence study in another year, say 1980, making sure to use the same methods and criteria as in the first study. If the age-specific DMF rates for 1980 are then plotted, the birth cohort with the low rate would be 50- to 54-year-olds, as illustrated in Figure 10.3. In this instance, the age cohort born in the 1926–1930 period has an unusually low DMF rate, indicating the possibility of exposure of this cohort to some protective effect early in life.

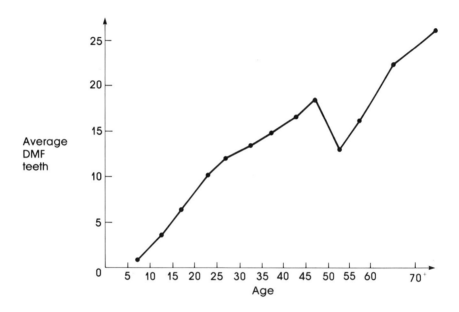

Figure 10.3 Average DMF for Black men, by age, North Carolina, 1980 (hypothetical).

Exercise 10.7

☐ What possible events or happenings could have produced this cohort effect?

Comment

The answer is now available because a repeat of the study did *not* confirm this suspected cohort effect. However, if the cohort effect had been confirmed—in this instance an unusually low rate—then clearly something happened to those born around 1926–1930 that protected them from caries and may do so until their death. One possibility worth consideration is that the Great Depression inculcated low candy-eating habits and other dietary practices promotive of good dental health. What other explanations can you suggest? It is interesting to speculate about possible explanations as to why no cohort effect was confirmed. We would have to consider all of our method pitfalls and test the data for their potential contribution to nonconfirmaton of the cohort hypothesis.

Exercise 10.8

☐ a. What should make us consider a cohort effect?

☐ b. What data do we need to establish an age (birth) cohort phenomenon?

Comment

a. Cohort effect is a possible explanation in cross-sectional studies or mortality data that show:

1. any association of a disease with age;

2. an unexpected dip or increase in the distribution of a disease by age (this may be shown by a bimodal distribution);

3. an unexpected secular decline in a nontreatable disease (for example, the considerable decline in deaths from cancer of the stomach over time in the United States, for which there is as yet no satisfactory explanation).

b. We need several cross-sectional studies at different times, each one by age with similar methods being used.

Note: The classic cohort analysis was that of Wade Hampton Frost, who studied tuberculosis mortality in Massachusetts in the 1930s. Consistently over time he identified a birth cohort that had higher rates of tuberculosis throughout their lives. We urge you to read his papers.[41]

Summary

The main points covered in Chapter 10 include:

1. The nature of cohorts.

2. Data needed to determine whether a birth cohort effect exists.

3. The findings that should make one suspect the possibility of a cohort effect.

4. Relevance of cohorts in interpreting data.

References and Further Reading Sources

Topic	Reference number	Pages
Cohort effect and birth cohort analysis	13	389–390
	27	60–63
	36	100–104
	38	186–190
	40	81–90
	41	593–600

Statistical Tests of Significance:
Putting Them in Their Correct Place

11

In previous chapters, we compared groups' rates of diseases or the means of health attributes such as blood pressure; such comparisons are the basics of epidemiology. We found differences, one group being higher or lower than the others, and made note of the need to exclude any effects due to sampling variability in interpreting these differences. Such exclusion requires tests of significance; they are statistical concepts and do not determine by themselves the biological, social, or "real life" meaning or importance of differences.

So in this chapter, we look more closely at differences in health status between groups and consider in more detail those mysterious "statistical tests of significance" that have been alluded to in previous chapters.

Exercise 11.1

The Table 11.1 was obtained from a hypothetical ten-year cohort study of a random sample of 2,000 men aged 40 to 49 to test the association of stroke and stress. By happenstance, our random sample of 2,000 men resulted in 1,000 "stressed" and 1,000 "nonstressed" men. Obviously, because it is a cohort study, all subjects were free from stroke at the start. Because we have a random sample of men free of stroke, the prevalence of stress in this population can be estimated from Table 11.1 as 1,000/2,000 = 0.50.

Table 11.1   **Male Subjects, Aged 40–49, by Stress Status at Beginning of Study and Stroke Status at End of Study**

	Stress status		
Stroke status	Stressed	Nonstressed	Total
Developed stroke	300	100	400
Did not develop stroke	700	900	1,600
Total	1,000	1,000	2,000

☐ a. What variables are controlled for in this study?

☐ b. What is the incidence, or risk, of stroke among the stressed group?

☐ c. What is the incidence, or risk, of stroke among the non-stressed group?

☐ d. What is the relative risk?

□ e. What is the attributable risk?

□ f. What is the population attributable risk percent (or etiologic fraction)?

Write down your answers, then read the discussions below. This is a chance to review some of the epidemiological terms and indices discussed in previous chapters.

Comment

a. Sex and age are controlled for by subject selection because all of the subjects are men 40 to 49 years old at the beginning of the study.

b. The incidence rate of stroke among stressed men is 300/1,000 = 0.30.

c. The incidence rate of stroke among nonstressed men is 100/1,000 = 0.10.

d. The relative risk is 0.30/.10 = 3.0.

e. Attributable risk (simple attributable risk) is 0.30 minus 0.10 = 0.20.

f. The population attributable risk percent (PARP) can be calculated (as you learned in Chapter 4) from the formula:

$$\frac{P(RR-1)}{P(RR-1)} \times 100$$

where *P* is the prevalence of the risk factor (in this instance, stress) in the population and *RR* is the relative risk for stressed men. Therefore, in this study,

$$\text{PARP} = \frac{0.50(3-1)}{0.50(3-1)+1} = \frac{1}{2} = 0.50, \text{or } 50\%$$

Because this a cohort study, we are able to estimate the attributable risk and therefore use it in the alternate formula: $PARP = P(AR)/RT$, where AR is the attributable risk, RT is the disease rate in the total sample, and P is the prevalence of the risk factor. Applying the data, we get $PARP = (0.50)(0.20)/0.20 = 0.50$, as before. It should not surprise you by now that the $PARP$ calculation is the same using either formula.

Remember, the data are hypothetical. Do not jump to any conclusions about the real association of stress with stroke.

Exercise 11.2

☐ Do the two calculated incidence rates differ from each other?

Comment

Yes, they surely do, since 0.30 and 0.10 differ from each other. From an epidemiological and practical viewpoint the difference is meaningful, too, in that the difference of 20% is a lot, particularly where the risk factor (stress) is common.

Exercise 11.3

☐ Can the difference found be an artifact due to any method pitfall that we learned about earlier? Why, or why not?

Comment

We need to consider these possible explanations before trying to interpret the process by which stress produces strokes in men. There is no sense in considering processes if the association is artifactual.

However, we do not know the answer from the table. Entities such as the validity of the diagnosis of stroke and the ways of classification of stress are not indicated here. Sex and age are not confounders, but your knowledge suggests that other potential confounders are not controlled for in this table. In particular, you know that blood pressure is associated with stress and with stroke, so that blood pressure may be creating an artifactual association between stroke and stress.

Exercise 11.4

When all confounding effects are eliminated, then one should consider the possibility of sampling variability producing this difference.

☐ Under what circumstances is sampling variability a relevant consideration?

Comment

Only when you have studied a *sample* can its variability be relevant.

Exercise 11.5

☐ If the 2,000 men were the entire population, would the difference in stroke incidence be real? Why or why not?

Comment

Yes, because the incidence rates are the actual population parameters and are not derived from samples. In reality, therefore, if the total population is included in a study, tests of significance are not necessary because no sampling variability is involved. In effect, the findings are not *estimates* of the truth (of the real parameters of the population) but the truth itself.

However, as in our hypothetical study of stress, entire populations of interest are not included in most research studies because they are usually too large, and it would be too costly and too time-consuming to include everybody. Therefore, a sample of the members of the population generally is used in studies.

Exercise 11.6

☐ a. Would you agree with the concept that "total" populations, even such as the world population, are samples of larger populations or samples of future populations from the same place, and that therefore even total populations should be regarded as samples?

☐ b. If you agree, would you therefore acknowledge that sampling variability applies in every study? Indicate why you think so.

Comment

a. This is a debatable notion, so any opinion you hold is likely to be shared by others. The true believers in this concept that all populations are samples claim that they wish always to apply the results of their current research to current or future populations similar to the one under study. Some opponents regard the concept as a way to provide employment for statisticians.

b. If you are a believer in this concept, then you would have to consider sampling variability in every study, even when the entire population is used. However, even disbelievers in this concept sometimes are forced by editors or reviewers of scientific publications into considering sampling variability in studies using entire populations. You will have to make up your own mind on this issue.

Exercise 11.7

☐ In this study, we know that the 2,000 men constitute a random sample of stressed and nonstressed men and, thus, the sample estimates reflect the population parameters. Can we then conclude that the population parameters differ from each other? Why or why not?

Comment

No, not yet. What *is* clear is that the incidence rates *in the two samples* do differ (0.10 and 0.30 are different). However, it is not known and will never be known whether the incidence rates in the two populations differ because all members of these two populations were not measured. We can estimate the parameters and therefore the difference, from the samples, but the estimates will vary with each sample drawn. If another sample of 1,000 stressed men and 1,000 nonstressed men had been selected, the two incidence rates might have turned out to be 0.15 for nonstressed and 0.28 for stressed men. Or if still another sample had been selected, the sample incidence rates might have been 0.09 and 0.31. Hence, the notion of variability produced by samples.

Exercise 11.8

☐ If, in fact, the parameters, the two population incidence rates, are exactly the same and if samples of 1,000 stressed and 1,000 nonstressed men are followed for ten years, would the sample incidence rates turn out to be the same? Why or why not?

Comment

Well, they *might*, but in general the answer is *no* because both sample incidence rates are subject to sampling variability. That is, each sample incidence rate may differ somewhat from the population parameter because a sample was measured rather than the entire population.

Thus, when two (or more) observed sample rates are compared to each other, they may differ only because of sampling variability *or* because of sampling variability *and* a difference between the population parameters. All statistical tests of significance address that issue, and that is their correct place in our epidemiological pursuits.

This idea is fundamental, so mull it over and be sure you understand it before proceeding.

Exercise 11.9

☐ What is the question or hypothesis addressed by this study?

Comment

One might say: "Stress is a risk factor for stroke." In this study, the researcher tests the working hypothesis that the incidence rate for stroke is greater among stressed men than among nonstressed men.

You are correct if you said something similar, but statisticians prefer us to express our hypotheses as if no differences were there, that is, in the null fashion, and then to set about disproving this null hypothesis by using a test of significance. The word "null" is derived from the Latin *nullus,* which means "none." In a sense, statisticians are saying that if we can disprove the nonexistence of an association, then we prove the existence of that association.

An illustrative analogy may be the legal notion of "not guilty" until proven otherwise. Our example may be extended to the fantasy court case that followed this hypothetical study when the defending lawyer for the stress industry pleaded "not guilty" to the damage suit brought by the stroke victims. In rejecting this plea of not guilty, the jury would find the stress industry guilty.

Thus, the no-guilt plea presumes that there is no association of stress with stroke in the population (the null hypothesis). In rejecting this plea, the jury must accept the opposite and rule that an association does exist.

Exercise 11.10

☐ In light of the need to keep statisticians happy, restate the hypothesis of this study in the null format.

Comment

The null hypothesis (H_o in statistical shorthand) is that the incidence rate of stroke in stressed men (one true parameter) is the same as the incidence rate of stroke in nonstressed men (the other true parameter).

In further shorthand, we can let IR_s and IR_{ns} be the population parameters, the incidence rates for stressed and nonstressed men, respectively. Thus, in shorthand the null hypothesis is written

$$H_o{:}IR_s = IR_{ns} \quad \text{or} \quad H_o{:} IR_s - IR_{ns} = 0$$

(which is why it is called "null").

Many studies, particularly descriptive epidemiological ones, do not specifically indicate any null hypotheses. However, the researchers reflect their null hypotheses implicitly in the comparisons they make. Most researchers state explicitly the hypotheses they wish to substantiate with their study data, for example, stress and stroke are related. This kind of hypothesis, expressing some sort of *inequality*, statisticians call the *alternate hypothesis*. Any null hypothesis and its corresponding alternate hypothesis should cover all possible situations in reality. Thus, if the null hypothesis is not true, then the alternate hypothesis must be true, and vice versa.

To avoid verbiage, statisticians use different symbols to distinguish between population parameters and estimates of these parameters from sample data. A common system that you will see in biostatistics textbooks and journal articles is to choose some symbol for the population parameter, such as IR, and then slap a "hat" (∧) on it to represent the sample estimate of that parameter, $\widehat{IR}$. This-funny looking fellow, IR, is called "IR hat."

Exercise 11.11

☐ a. If the null hypothesis *is* true, what would you *expect* the difference to be between $\widehat{IR}_s$ and $\widehat{IR}_{ns}$? (Remember, these are sample estimates.)

□ b. If the null hypothesis *is not* true, what would you *expect* the difference to be between $\widehat{IR}_s$ and $\widehat{IR}_{ns}$?

Comment

a. The difference would be expected to be close to zero. Sampling variability is likely to keep the difference from being exactly equal to zero.

b. The difference would be expected to be quite different from zero. It is produced by sampling variability *and* by the differences in the population parameters.

Exercise 11.12

Now, let us reverse the logic of the previous thought.

□ a. If the observed difference between $\widehat{IR}_s$ and $\widehat{IR}_{ns}$ is close to zero or very small, would you reject the null hypothesis? State reasons.

□ b. If the observed difference between $\widehat{IR}$, and $\widehat{IR}_{ns}$ is large, would you reject the null hypothesis? State reasons.

Comment

a. No. If the difference is close to zero, it seems likely that this difference is due *only* to sampling variability, indicating that the null hypothesis is not false (it is true).

b. Yes. If the difference is large, it seems likely that the difference is not caused *only* by sampling variability, indicating that the null hypothesis is false.

Exercise 11.13

☐ But what is "very small" and what is "large" in regard to differences? Do we just make up numbers, or is there some rational basis for deciding when a difference is large enough to allow us to reject the null hypothesis?

Comment

There must be some rational basis; we do *not* pluck numbers out of our heads. An appropriately chosen test of significance lets you calculate the probability of obtaining a difference between sample estimates as large as the observed difference, *given* that the null hypothesis is true. If the calculated probability is large, it means that the difference between these estimates was likely to occur if the null hypothesis were true. If, however, the probability turns out to be small, it means that the difference between the sample estimates was unlikely to occur under the assumption that the null hypothesis is true, that is, because of sampling variability *only*. Hence, you would probably reject the null hypothesis with that degree of probability.

This calculated probability is often called a "p-value" and denoted by "p" (because p is the first letter of the word probability). Now you can understand the relevance of those mysterious "p's" when you see them in research articles.

Exercise 11.14

Let us consider two possibilities with the stress/stroke example used here. Recall that the two incidence rates are 0.30 and 0.10.

☐ a. Suppose a p-value of 0.50 is calculated by the test of significance. Would you reject your null hypothesis? Why or why not?

☐ b. If the p-value were 0.002 instead of 0.50, would you come to the same conclusion? Why or why not?

Comment

a. No, because the chances are 50–50 that a difference as large as 0.20 could occur due only to sampling variability when the null hypothesis is true. Thus, you would conclude that the population parameters IR_s and IR_{ns} do not differ.

b. No. Chances are only 2 out of 1,000 that a difference as large as 0.20 would be found due only to sampling variability if the null hypothesis were true. Thus, you would reject the null hypothesis and conclude that the population parameters IR_s and IR_{ns} do differ.

Exercise 11.15

When you use a test of significance to decide whether or not to reject a null hypothesis, it is possible for you to err in either of two directions. You can (a) disagree with something that is true or (b) fail to disagree (agree) with something that is false.

☐ Describe these two kinds of errors in terms of the null hypothesis.

Comment

a. One error is that you reject the null hypothesis when it is really true. Researchers call this a **Type I error.**

b. Another error is that you fail to reject a null hypothesis that is false. This is called a **Type II error.**

Returning to the hypothetical "stress industry" on trial will illustrate these two types of errors. On one hand, if stress is not associated with stroke (the null hypothesis is true) and the jury finds the stress industry guilty (it rejects the null hypothesis), then the jury has made a Type I error. On the other hand, if stress is associated with stroke (the null hypothesis is false) and the jury finds the stress industry not guilty (it does not reject the null hypothesis), then the jury has made a Type II error.

Do not get too dismayed. It is possible to make *correct* decisions, too, by using tests of significance. You can be correct in your decisions when you reject a null hypothesis when it is false and fail to reject a null hypothesis when it is true.

Exercise 11.16

Perhaps now is a good time for you to come up with a way of remembering the distinction between the two types of errors.

☐ Try one way for yourself—be it a limerick, mnemonic, anecdote or whatever—before looking at our suggestion. Write it down here.

Comment

Any way that works for you is fine. Table 11.2 shows one you might use. In reality, the null hypothesis is either true or not true. Your decision as a result of doing a test of significance is either to reject the null hypothesis or not. The table illustrates the four possible outcomes. The two cells marked "OK" illustrate a decision that corresponds to reality. The other two cells show the two types of errors.

Table 11.2   Distinguishing Between Type I and Type II Errors

Your decision as a result of a test of significance	Reality	
	H_o true	H_o not true
Reject H_o	Type I error	OK (correct decision)
Do not reject H_o	OK (correct decision)	Type II error

Exercise 11.17

☐ Using your method or our table, it will be easy for you to answer the following question. If you reject the null hypothesis, do you know for certain that the null hypothesis is false? Why or why not?

Comment

Unfortunately, no. The null hypothesis could be false, but it is also possible that you could be making a Type I error. Obviously, good researchers do not like to make errors, so they try to minimize the possibility of doing so. When doing a test of significance, researchers choose for themselves the maximum probability of making a Type I error that they are willing to tolerate. This is called the size of their Type I error and is often denoted by the Greek symbol α (pronounced **"alpha"**). Statisticians often use Greek letters to denote statistical concepts, maybe because the Greeks were famous mathematicians.

Exercise 11.18

☐ Well, if that is the case, why not choose α or your α-level to be equal to zero and avoid making a Type I error at all?

Comment

Good try, but it will not work because the test of significance will tell you *never* to reject the null hypothesis—that is how the test of significance avoids making a Type I error at all. With the size of the Type I error equal to zero, you do not need to do the study because, no matter what the data look like, the test of significance will never reject the null hypothesis.

Since most researchers *want* to reject the null hypothesis in order to prove their point, they choose some nonzero value, usually a low one, for α and just live with that degree of error. A common choice for the size of Type I error is 0.05, but there is nothing magical about its use. You could just as well choose 0.10 or 0.08 or 0.03 for your α-level.

Exercise 11.19

☐ If you do not reject the null hypothesis, do you know for certain that the null hypothesis is true? Why or why not?

Comment

Unfortunately again, the answer is no, because you could be making a Type II error.

Researchers do not like to make Type II errors either. Unlike the size of the Type I error, which the researcher chooses fairly arbitrarily, the size of the Type II error is influenced by three components of the study: (1) sample size, (2) the chosen level of Type I error, and (3) the size of the difference between the population parameters.

The size of the Type II error is often denoted by β (pronounced **"beta"**), another of those Greek letters statisticians love. The larger the sample size, the smaller the sampling variability and, thus, the smaller the Type II error (β). The smaller the size of the Type I error, the larger the Type II error (the smaller α is, the larger β is). The greater the difference between the population parameters, the smaller the size of Type II error.

That is why, in planning a good study, you first choose your desired size of Type I error knowing that it will influence the size of the Type II error. Then you get some idea of the size of the expected difference between the population parameters you are studying; this information can be obtained from other published studies or from your own pretest. Then, specifying a tolerable size for Type II error, and using the help of a statistician or statistical tables, you can determine how large your sample needs to be in order to meet your specifications. If the needed sample size turns out to be larger than you can afford to include in your study, then you will have to settle for a larger size of Type I error or a larger size of Type II error.

It should be obvious to you that the *size* of a sample does not determine whether you can relate your findings to a population, that is, make generalizations from your sample. In order to make such generalizations, the sample (whether small or large) must truly represent the population, which is why considerable care needs to be taken in your study in the way you select your sample. Clearly, all of these choices require deliberation, and it is wise to include the aid of a statistician or a statistical textbook in this process.

In reality, you will see many studies in which the researcher has not considered the interrelationship of size of Type I and Type II errors, size of sample, and expected differences between the population parameters.

Exercise 11.20

To put this all in perspective, suppose you have chosen your α-level and β-level and determined the necessary sample size for your expected difference in the population parameters. Having completed your study and applied the appropriate test of significance to your data, you will end up with a p-value.

☐ a. What is the interpretation of the p-value?

□ b. If the p-value is 0.01 and your chosen α-level is 0.05, what are you able to infer about the null hypothesis?

□ c. If the p-value is 0.17 and your chosen α-level is 0.10, what are you able to infer about the null hypothesis?

Comment

a. The p-value is the *probability* you would obtain a difference in sample estimates as large as the difference you got *if* the null hypothesis were true. Alternately, the p-value is the probability that the sample estimates differ only because of sampling variability.

b. Because your p-value is less than your chosen size of Type I error, you will reject the null hypothesis. That is, the probability is 1 in 100 that you would obtain the difference in sample estimates you did *if* the null hypothesis is true. Therefore, the probability that you will be making a Type I error in rejecting the null hypothesis is tolerable.

c. Reasoning as in (b), you will not reject the null hypothesis because your p-value is greater than your α-level.

Your understanding of these concepts and their place in epidemiology permits you to read scientific articles and realize that these concepts often are used incorrectly and/or inappropriately. Many such articles or scientific presentations do not explicate these concepts. For example, the null hypothesis may never be stated, although it is always implied, and no concern about the size of Type II error is evident. Also, the chosen α level may not be stated but, rather, only the p-value may be reported Researchers often do not report the exact p-values and give some indication of how small it is by writing p<0.01 or p<0.05 or p<0.001, and so forth.

Some researchers attempt to rate the relative *importance* of their data in terms of the size of the p-value by believing that a smaller p-value indicates more importance. That is why you will read terms such as "highly significant," "very highly significant," "approaching significance," and "almost significant." This practice should not be encouraged, we believe, because the size of the p-value has no relationship to the potential practical significance of the findings. Further reading about these concepts can be found in the references included at the end of this chapter.

Summary

This chapter covered the following:

1. A statistical test of significance tells you whether or not sample estimates differ only because of sampling variability.

2. The format of a test of significance is to reject or not reject a null hypothesis.

3. One can make two possible kinds of errors in performing a test of significance—a Type I error and a Type II error.

4. The design of a study should include specification of the acceptable sizes for Type I and Type II errors, the expected difference between the population parameters, and the necessary sample size to attain these acceptable levels.

5. You decide whether or not to reject the null hypothesis by comparing your α-level with the p-value obtained from the test of significance.

6. Regardless of the foregoing, the nature of the sample *and not the p-value* will determine whether you are able to make inferences to the population of interest. In order to make such inferences, clearly the sample must be representative of the population.

References and Further Reading Sources

Topic	Reference number	Pages
Statistical tests of significance	16	1–7
	24	285–334
	27	28
	29	1–13
	29	309–312
Types I and II errors	16	115–123
	53	163–167
	53	239–240
Null hypothesis	34	201–203
	53	166–167

Types of Data and the Chi Square Test

12

In the previous chapter, we learned about statistical tests of significance and their place in epidemiological research. In Chapter 12, we take a look at the sorts of variables used and the numerical or mathematical properties of these variables. The types of variables we use determine what statistical techniques we can apply to describe population parameters and also determine which is the appropriate statistical test of significance to use.

Exercise 12.1

Variables or characteristics that are used often in epidemiology because of their association with many diseases include age, sex, ethnic group, marital status, and social class.

☐ In what way do the variables age and sex differ as far as their numerical properties are concerned?

Write down your answer, then read the following discussion.

Comment

Age has a number associated with it, for example, 35 years old. Sex, however, has no number associated with it but is simply "named" male or female.

Exercise 12.2

☐ Many researchers distinguish between *quantitative* and *qualitative* variables. Decide for age and sex whether the variable is quantitative or qualitative.

Comment

Age is **quantitative** because it is measured in terms of "how much of" the variable age you have.

Sex, on the other hand, is a **qualitative** variable. The label male or female simply describes what sex you are; there is no attempt to measure "how much" of the variable sex you have. Qualitative variables are also called **nominal variables** because the different values of the variables are simply names. Qualitative variables are also called **categorical variables** because the different values of the variable indicate categories into which persons can be classified.

Exercise 12.3

☐ Now that you know that age is quantitative and sex is qualitative (or nominal or categorical), what implications does this have for the types of statistical techniques you might use on these two variables?

Comment

Because age is a quantitative variable, you can calculate the average age (arithmetic mean) of a group of people. Because sex is not a quantitative variable, it makes no sense to calculate an average sex; you can simply report the proportion (or rate) of persons in a group that is female and the proportion that is male.

Sometimes in coding data for research studies, the different values of the qualitative variables are coded with numbers because usually it is easier for computers to read numbers than words. For example, marital status is a qualitative variable: "never married" may be coded as 1, "currently married" as 2, "divorced" as 3, "separated" as 4, and "widowed" as 5. Although it may appear that marital status is now a quantitative variable, it really is not, and it would be pure folly to average together the numerical values for marital status and obtain an average marital status.

Exercise 12.4

☐ Consider the variable "self-perceived health status" rated on a four-point scale from excellent, good, fair, to poor. How does this variable differ on its numerical properties from a nominal variable like marital status and from a quantitative variable like age?

Comment

Self-perceived health status may appear at first glance to be a nominal variable (because its values are named excellent, good, fair, and poor), but it differs from marital status in that the different values of health status are ordered. Excelient health is better than good health, fair health is better than poor health, and so forth. There is no implicit ordering among the different values for marital statuses, regardless of your opinion about them, or among the different values for *any* nominal variable. For this reason, variables like self-perceived health status, which have an order to them, are called **ordinal variables.**

Although self-perceived health status does have an "order" about it, there is no way to measure exactly the "quantity" of health like we can measure age (or weight or height or number of teeth). Some researchers apply numbers to the values on the ordinal scale: 4 = excellent, 3 = good, fair = 2, and poor = 1, and then proceed to calculate a mean (average) self-perceived health status. Calculating a mean from these numbers is valid only if the differences between the numbers reflect actual differences between the levels of health. For example, the difference between excellent and good is 1 (4-3) and, also, the difference between good and fair is 1 (3-2). Hence, the numbers applied to this scale assume that the difference between excellent and good is the same as the difference between good and fair.

Some researchers do not make the assumption that the ordered values of the ordinal variable correspond to some numerical quantity of the variable. Rather, they use statistical techniques for ordered or ranked data; these techniques are called nonparametric statistics, as opposed to parametric statistics, which are applicable to quantitative data.

It is obvious that a quantitative variable, such as age, is used often as an ordinal variable (for example, age categories such as 20–29, 30–39, or 40–49) or as a nominal variable (old versus young). If age is used as a nominal variable, then it should be considered to be a nominal variable for that study.

Exercise 12.5

So we have three different types of variables: qualitative (or nominal or categorical), ordinal, and quantitative. Recall that some researchers measure ordinal variables, assign numerical quantities to the values of the variable, and then pretend that the variable is quantitative.

□ Consider now the two quantitative variables "number of children ever born" and "weight." How do these two variables differ as far as their numerical properties are concerned?

Comment

"Number of children ever born" can only assume a value such as 0, 2, 13, or 5. It cannot asume a value like 3.02 or 3.27. However, "weight" can assume the value 105 pounds or 105.2 pounds or 105.23 pounds, depending upon the accuracy of the scale in measuring weight.

These two kinds of quantitative variables are called *discrete* and *continuous*. A discrete quantitative variable, like "number of children ever born," can assume only a limited number of values. A continuous quantitative variable, like weight, can assume an infinite number of possible values.

Averages or means are obtained for both discrete and continuous variables, but they have somewhat different interpretations. When an average weight of 105.37 pounds is reported, it certainly is possible for someone in that group to weigh exactly 105.37 pounds. However, when the average number of children ever born is reported to be 2.1, it certainly is not possible for anyone in that group to have had 2.1 children. Although it is appropriate to obtain averages for both discrete and continuous variables, one needs to be careful of interpretation.

Exercise 12.6

Knowing the type of variables you have in your study will allow you also to decide which statistical tests of significance may be appropriate for your study. Let us go back to the example of the possible relationship between stress and stroke, which was discussed in Chapter 11.

□ What are the independent and dependent variables in this example? Are they nominal, ordinal, or quantitative?

Comment

The independent variable is presence or absence of stress and it is a nominal variable. (Note that it might also be considered an ordinal variable because people with stress have more of it than people without stress. However, when there are only two possible ordered values of the variable, as in this case, it is usually considered nominal rather than ordinal.)

The dependent variable is presence or absence of a stroke over some defined time period. This is a nominal variable also.

This example illustrates a very common research design in epidemiology—the investigation of the relationship between two nominal variables. Often the independent variable is the presence or absence of the characteristic and the dependent variable is the presence or absence of the disease. The statistical test of significance that assesses whether or not the observed differences between rates in this study design are due only to sampling variability is called a **chi square** (χ^2) **test.** (The symbol χ is "chi"; it is pronounced "kigh," which rhymes with "high.")

Exercise 12.7

Let us do a test of significance for the stress/stroke example we have been discussing. The data from this cohort study are shown in Table 12.1 (remember they are hypothetical data).

Table 12.1   ***Frequency of Male Subjects, Aged 40–49 by
Stress Status at Beginning of Study and Stroke Status
at End of Study***

| | Stress status | | |
Stroke status	Stressed	Nonstressed	Total
Developed stroke	300	100	400
Did not develop stroke	700	900	1,600
Total	1,000	1,000	2,000

☐ a. What is the null hypothesis?

☐ b. Basically, what sample statistics are going to be compared?
All of this should be an easy review from Chapter 11.

Comment

a. Using the notation from Chapter 11, the null hypothesis
is H_o: $IR_s = IR_{ns}$ This is equivalent to stating that the incidence rate for
stroke is "independent of" or "not associated with" or "not related to"
presence of stress.

b. The sample proportions or incidence rates $\widehat{IR}_s$ and $\widehat{IR}_{ns}$, which equal 0.30 and 0.10, respectively, will be compared.

Exercise 12.8

In order to arrive at the p-value, it is necessary to calculate a test statistic that quantifies the difference between the observed outcome (the data in Table 12.1) and the outcome one would expect if the null hypothesis is true. Let us see how this works.

□ What numerical values for the sample incidence rates would be expected, *assuming* the null hypothesis to be true?

Comment

If the null hypothesis is true, then the sample incidence rates would be relatively close to each other and would differ only because of sampling variability. What value would they be? That is a more difficult question. If you knew what the incidence of stroke is in 40- to 49-year-old men, then that information might be used to specify the expected sample incidence rates. Usually, though, such information is not available.

Thus, in most cases it is necessary to use the sample data itself to estimate what the sample incidence rates would be if the null hypothesis is true. Under this assumption, all 2,000 persons in the sample would be at the same risk of stroke. The data indicate that 400 of these persons developed a stroke. Hence, an estimate of the common incidence rate or overall rate, if the null hypothesis is true, is 400/2,000 or 0.20.

Exercise 12.9

☐ a. Using the overall incidence rate of 0.20, which assumes the null hypothesis to be true, how many of the 1,000 stressed persons and how many of the 1,000 nonstressed persons would be expected to develop a stroke?

☐ b. How many of the 1,000 subjects in each group would be expected *not* to develop a stroke, assuming the null hypothesis to be true?

Comment

a. The calculation is the same for each group: $(1,000) \times (0.20)$ = 200. Therefore, one would expect 200 of the stressed and 200 of the nonstressed to develop a stroke, if the null hypothesis is true.

b. If 200 per group are expected to suffer a stroke, then 800 per group $(1,000 - 200)$ would be expected *not* to suffer a stroke.

Exercise 12.10

Consider now the four "cells" in Table 12.2, stressed with stroke, nonstressed with stroke, stressed without stroke, and nonstressed without stroke. Compare the expected number of subjects (abbreviated as *E*) with the observed number of subjects (abbreviated as *O*) in each of the four cells. The observed number of subjects is simply the information from Table 12.1 and the expected number of subjects was calculated in Exercise 12.9

Table 12.2   *Observed and Expected Subjects, by Stress Status and by Stroke Status*

	Stress status		
Stroke status	Stressed	Nonstressed	Total
Developed stroke	O = 300 E = 200	O = 100 E = 200	400
Did not develop stroke	O = 700 E = 800	O = 900 E = 800	1,600
Total	1,000	1,000	2,000

☐ If the null hypothesis is true, what would be the relationship between the observed number of subjects and the expected number of subjects per cell?

Comment

The observed number and expected number of subjects per cell probably would be relatively close to each other. But, we also know they would differ somewhat due to sampling variability.

The χ^2 statistic quantifies the amount of discrepancy between the observed and expected number of subjects per cell in the following manner. For each cell, the difference between the observed number of subjects and expected number of subjects is calculated. This is denoted by $(O_j - E_j)$, where the subscript j refers to a particular cell. Some of the values of $(O_j - E_j)$ will be positive and some will be negative. In order to have a measure of discrepancy that is never negative, the quantity $(O_j - E_j)$ is squared, or multiplied by itself $(O_j - E_j)^2$. Further, because a larger difference between O_j and E_j is likely to occur the larger the value of E_j, the squared difference is adjusted for the size of E_j by dividing by E_j; that is, $(O_j - E_j)^2/E_j$.

This quantity or ratio is calculated for each of the four cells in Table 12.2. The sum of these four quantities then is the χ^2 statistic, which quantifies the amount of discrepancy between the observed number of subjects and the expected number of subjects.

Exercise 12.11

☐ For each cell in Table 12.2, calculate $(O_j - E_j)^2/E_j$. Then add up these four quantities to obtain the χ^2 statistic.

Comment

For the stressed/stroke cell, we have $(300 - 200)^2/200 = (100)^2/200 = 10{,}000/200 = 50.0$.

For the nonstressed/stroke cell, we have $(100 - 200)^2/200 = (-100)^2/200 = 10{,}000/200 = 50.0$. Recall that $(-100) \times (-100) = +10{,}000$.

For the stressed/nonstroke cell, we have $(700 - 800)^2/800 = 10,000/800 = 12.50$.

For the nonstressed/nonstroked cell, we have the equation $(900 - 800)^2/800 = 10,000/800 = 12.50$.

Adding these four quantities, we obtain $\chi^2 = 125.0$.

Exercise 12.12

Consider a χ^2 statistic calculated from any 2×2 table, like Table 12.2.

☐ a. What are the smallest and largest possible values that the χ^2 statistic could possibly assume?

☐ b. If the null hypothesis is true, what sort of values of the χ^2 statistic would one expect to obtain?

☐ c. If the null hypothesis is not true, what sort of values of the χ^2 statistic would one expect to obtain?

Comment

a. The smallest possible value for the χ^2 statistic is zero. This would occur only if the expected number equals the observed number of subjects in every single cell. The largest possible value could approach infinity.

b. If the null hypothesis is true, then the expected number and observed number of subjects per cell should be fairly close, any variation resulting only from sampling variability. Hence, the resulting χ^2 statistic should be fairly small, but not exactly equal to zero, although a χ^2 statistic summed over a large table with many cells would probably be larger than a χ^2 statistic summed over a smaller table with fewer cells.

c. If the null hypothesis is false, then the value of the χ^2 statistic should be large, since a false null hypothesis will result in larger discrepancies between the expected number and observed number of subjects per cell.

Over the years, statisticians have studied the χ^2 distribution and have provided us with tables that allow us to make probability statements about the χ^2 statistic. Using these tables, we can figure out the probability that we would obtain a χ^2 statistic as large as or larger than the one we obtained in our study, *if* the null hypothesis is true (if there is no association). Table 12.3 gives an abbreviated table of the χ^2 distribution, which is sufficient for most researchers' purposes.

Actually, there are several different χ^2 distributions, each one depending upon how many quantities were added together to obtain the χ^2 statistic. (In our stress/stroke example, four quantities were added to obtain our χ^2 statistic.)

Each of the different χ^2 probability distributions is specified by a quantity called its **"degrees of freedom,"** abbreviated as df. In Table 12.3, the "degrees of freedom" is denoted by df and each line of Table 12.3 gives the probability distribution for a particular χ^2 distribution defined by its df.

Exercise 12.13

☐ How many different χ^2 distributions are contained in Table 12.3 and what are the different values of the df?

Table 12.3   Upper Percentage Points of the χ² Distribution

a = .10	a = .05	a = .025	a = .010	a = .005	df
2.70554	3.84146	5.02389	6.63490	7.87944	1
4.60517	5.99147	7.37776	9.21034	10.5966	2
6.25139	7.81473	9.34840	11.3449	12.8381	
7.77944	9.48773	11.1433	13.2767	14.8602	4
9.23635	11.0705	12.8325	15.0863	16.7496	5
10.6446	12.5916	14.4494	16.8119	18.5476	6
12.0170	14.0671	16.0128	18.4753	20.2777	7
13.3616	15.5073	17.5346	20.0902	21.9550	8
14.6837	16.9190	19.0228	21.6660	23.5893	9
15.9871	18.3070	20.4831	23.2093	25.1882	10
17.2750	19.6751	21.9200	24.7250	26.7569	11
18.5494	21.0261	23.3367	26.2170	28.2995	12
19.8119	22.3621	24.7356	27.6883	29.8194	13
21.0642	23.6848	26.1190	29.1413	31.3193	14
22.3072	24.9958	27.4884	30.5779	32.8013	15
23.5418	26.2962	28.8454	31.9999	34.2672	16
24.7690	27.5871	30.1910	33.4087	35.7185	17
25.9894	28.8693	31.5264	34.8053	37.1564	18
27.2036	30.1435	32.8523	36.1908	38.5822	19
28.4120	31.4104	34.1696	37.5662	39.9968	20
29.6151	32.6705	35.4789	38.9321	41.4010	21
30.8133	33.9244	36.7807	40.2894	42.7956	22
32.0069	35.1725	38.0757	41.6384	44.1813	23
33.1963	36.4151	39.3641	42.9798	45.5585	24
34.3816	37.6525	40.6465	44.3141	46.9278	25
35.5631	38.8852	41.9232	45.6417	48.2899	26
36.7412	40.1133	43.1944	46.9630	49.6449	27
37.9159	41.3372	44.4607	48.2782	50.9933	28
39.0875	42.5569	45.7222	49.5879	52.3356	29
40.2560	43.7729	46.9792	50.8922	53.6720	30
51.8050	55.7585	59.3417	63.6907	66.7659	40
63.1671	67.5048	71.4202	76.1539	79.4900	50
74.3970	79.0819	83.2976	88.3794	91.9517	60
85.5271	90.5312	95.0231	100.425	104.215	70
96.5782	101.879	106.629	112.329	116.321	80
107.565	113.145	118.136	124.116	128.299	90
118.498	124.342	129.561	135.807	140.169	100

Source: Tables of the percentage points of the χ²-distribution, *Biometrika* 32 188–189, by Catherine M. Thompson. Reproduced by permission of the *Biometrika* Trustees.

Comment

Note that the column that denotes the "degrees of freedom" is the right-hand column. There are 37 different χ^2 distributions in Table 12.3, and the degrees of freedom are 1, 2, 3, . . . , 29, 30, 40, 50, 60, 70, 80, 90, 100.

Exercise 12.14

For Table 12.2, let us find the df for the χ^2 statistic. One way to figure out the df in tables such as Table 12.2 is to use a general formula:

degrees of freedom = (number columns − 1) × (number rows − 1)

where the number of columns and number of rows refer to the table under consideration.

☐ In Table 12.2, what would be the degrees of freedom?

Comment

Degrees of freedom = one because number of columns is two (stressed and nonstressed) and number of rows is two (developed a stroke and did not develop a stroke). Note that the product of the number of rows and columns (2 × 2 = 4 in this example) is the number of cells added to obtain the χ^2 statistic. (Note: Do *not* count the "total" column and "total" row as one of the rows or columns when you use this formula for df.)

The concept "degrees of freedom" also has an intuitive interpretation; it is the number of cells in the table whose expected number of subjects does not depend upon the expected number of subjects in other cells. For instance, in the cell "stressed and stroke" in Table 12.2, it was determined that 200 subjects would be expected in that cell if the null hypothesis were true. Given that, the expected number of subjects in the cell "stressed and no stroke" needs to be 800, because there are only a total number of 1,000 stressed persons in the study and 200 and 800 must add up to 1,000. Likewise, because it is given that 400 persons out of the total sample size of 2,000 developed a stroke, and it was calculated that 200 of these would be expected in the stressed group, then it is determined that 200 subjects must be expected in the "nonstressed and stroke" cell. Similarly, 800 subjects must be expected in the "nonstressed and no stroke" cell, because there must be a total of 1,000 nonstressed persons.

Thus, once one expected number is calculated for any cell in the table, the expected numbers in the remaining three cells are automatically determined due to the fixed marginal totals in the table (1,000 stressed, 1,000 nonstressed, 400 who developed a stroke, 1,600 who did not develop a stroke). Because there is only one cell whose expected value does not depend upon expected values in other cells, the df = 1.

You can illustrate for yourself that it does not matter which one of the four cells is selected to make the first calculation of expected number of subjects by choosing first the cell "stressed and did not develop a stroke" and then calculating the expected number of subjects for each cell.

Exercise 12.15

Consider the χ^2 distribution with df equal to one, the first line of Table 12.3. The columns of Table 12.3 are selected probability levels. For example, looking in the column marked .10 and the row labeled 1, one reads the number 2.70554. This is interpreted in the following manner: Given that the null hypothesis is true, the probability is .10 that a χ^2 variable with 1 degree of freedom will be 2.70554 or larger. That is, a value of 2.70554 or larger for a χ^2 variable with one degree of freedom is a somewhat unlikely event under the assumption that the null hypothesis is true.

   □ Write a statement to interpret the number 6.635 which is in the column labeled .010 and the row labeled 1 in Table 12.3.

Comment

Given that the null hypothesis is true, the probability is 0.01 that a x^2 variable with one degree of freedom will be 6.635 or larger. Hence, if a calculated x^2 statistic with 1 df is equal to 6.635, the p-value corresponding to this 6.635 is 0.01.

Exercise 12.16

□ Given that the calculated x^2 statistic for the stress/stroke example is 125.0, and given that it has one degree of freedom, use Table 12.3 to calculate a p-value. That is, what is the probability that the x^2 statistic, with one degree of freedom, would be as large as 125.0, or larger, given that the null hypothesis is true?

Comment

In Table 12.3, look along row 1 (df = one) for a number in the table close to 125.0. The closest available is 7.879. Hence, the p-value being sought here is not in Table 12.3, but it is known that the p-value is less than 0.005. Why? Because the probability is 0.005 that a x^2 variable with df = 1 will be as large as or larger than 7.879 if the null hypothesis is true. Because larger values of the χ^2 variable are *more unlikely* under the null hypothesis, the p-value corresponding to a value of 125.0 must be smaller than 0.005 (sometimes written as p<0.005).

Exercise 12.17

☐ a. If an alpha level (or size of Type I error) of 0.05 is being used for this statistical test of significance, and the p-value is less than 0.005, will the null hypothesis be rejected?

☐ b. What is the conclusion about stress and stroke?

Comment

a. Because the p-value, whatever it is, is less than 0.005, it must be less than 0.05. Therefore, the null hypothesis is rejected.

b. Rejection of the null hypothesis means that the incidence rates of stroke are not the same in the stressed and nonstressed populations. Because the sample incidence rate is higher in the stressed group, the further conclusion can be drawn that the incidence of stroke is higher in that population.

The χ^2 test just discussed for tables with two rows and two columns (called 2 × 2 contingency tables) is appropriate *only if* all four cells have their expected number of observations equal to or larger than five. This condition was met in Table 12.2. If this condition is *not* met, another statistical test of significance, called Fisher's Exact Test for 2 × 2 tables, can be used. This is an example of needing to know the assumptions of a statistical test so that you use it only in appropriate situations.

A note to statistical sophisticates: Those with a little biostatistical background may have noted that the χ^2 example we just did was a *two-sided* or *two-tailed* χ^2 test of significance. This simply means that our alternate hypothesis allowed for the possibility that the null hypothesis could be false in one of *two* possible ways—$IR_s > IR_{ns}$ or $IR_s < IR_{ns}$. The data, of course, indicated that the null hypothesis was false in the direction $IR_s > IR_{ns}$. Some people would argue a priori (before data are collected) that it is inconceivable or impossible that the null hypothesis would be false in the direction $IR_s < IR_{ns}$. These people would do a *one-sided* or *one-tailed* χ^2 test of significance, assuming that the null hypothesis could only be false in the direction $IR_s > IR_{ns}$. The χ^2 statistic would be calculated the same way as in our example. However, the p-value would be calculated slightly differently, resulting in a smaller p-value. Because the same empirical data yield a smaller p-value for a one-sided test than for a two-sided test, many researchers prefer to do a one-sided test when comparing two groups because they often want to reject the null hypothesis. However, one needs to be absolutely certain, a priori, that the null hypothesis could be false in only one possible direction. Those who like to "play it safe" usually choose to do a two-sided test.

Good discussions of the χ^2 statistic and its use are given in the references at the end of this chapter.

Exercise 12.18

Tests for association of two variables need not be done only in 2 × 2 contingency tables. Tables with more rows and columns can be used if appropriate. Consider now a slight modification of the stress and stroke study discussed in this chapter. Instead of classifying subjects as stressed or nonstressed, expand the classification to three levels; nonstressed, mildly stressed, and highly stressed. Assume that there is a random sample of 150 nonstressed, 100 mildly stressed, and 100 highly stressed—all males. The outcome of this cohort study is given in Table 12.4.

Table 12.4   *Male Subjects, by Stress Status and Stroke Status*

| | Stress status | | | |
Stroke status	None	Mild	High	Total
Developed a stroke	20	20	30	70
Did not develop a stroke	<u>130</u>	<u>80</u>	<u>70</u>	<u>280</u>
Total	150	100	100	350

☐ a. Write down the null hypothesis that the statistical test of significance will test.

☐ b. Calculate the value of the χ^2 statistic.

□ c. How many df does the χ^2 statistic have?

□ d. Find the p-value for your χ^2 statistic.

□ e. Using $\alpha = 0.05$, do you reject the null hypothesis? Why?

Comment

a. Using notation similar to that in Chapter 11, the null hypothesis is: H_o: $IR_{ns} = IR_{ms} = IR_{hs}$, where IR denotes incidence rate for stroke over some period and ns, ms, and hs mean nonstress, mild stress, and high stress, respectively.

b. Your table for observed and expected number of subjects per cell should be as in Table 12.5. The calculated value for the χ^2 statistic is 10.41. This was obtained as follows:

$$\frac{(20-30)^2}{30} + \frac{(20-20)^2}{20} + \frac{(30-20)^2}{20} + \frac{(130-120)^2}{120}$$
$$+ \frac{(80-80)^2}{80} + \frac{(70-80)^2}{80}$$

$$= 100\left(\frac{1}{30} + \frac{1}{20} + \frac{1}{120} + \frac{1}{80}\right)$$

$$= 100 \ (0.0333 + 0.0500 + 0.0083 + 0.0125)$$

$$= 100 \ (0.1041) = 10.41$$

**Table 12.5   Expected and Observed Subjects,
by Stress Status and Stroke Status**

	Stress status			
Stroke status	None	Mild	High	Total
Developed stroke	$O = 20$	$O = 20$	$O = 30$	
	$E = 30$	$E = 20$	$E = 20$	70
Did not develop stroke	$O = 130$	$O = 80$	$O = 70$	
	$E = 120$	$E = 80$	$E = 80$	280
Total	150	100	100	350

c. Using the formula (rows $-$ 1) $\times$ (columns $-$ 1) yields $(2 - 1) \times (3 - 1) = (1) \times (2) = 2$. Or recall from calculating the expected number of subjects per cell that there were two cells for which the expected number needed to be actually calculated, and then the expected number of subjects for the remaining four cells was immediately determined because the marginal totals were fixed. Hence, df = two.

d. Looking at row two of Table 12.3, for df = 2, a χ^2 value of 10.41 is not found. However, 10.41 is between 9.2 (which corresponds to a p-value of 0.01) and 10.6 (which corresponds to a p-value of 0.005). Hence, the p-value corresponding to $\chi^2 = 10.41$ is somewhere between 0.005 and .01.

e. Because the p-value is less than 0.01, the null hypothesis is rejected. The inference is that the incidence rates for stroke are not the same in all three stress populations. However, they could be "unequal" in a variety of ways. For example, the nonstressed could have a low incidence rate, whereas mildly and heavily stressed could have exactly the same incidence rate but higher than the nonstressed. Or all three incidence rates could differ from each other. You can think of other logical possiblities. The χ^2 statistic just calculated does not indicate which of these various situations is the case; additional statistical techniques need to be used to address this issue.

Many researchers, when obtaining a significant χ^2 statistic such as the 10.41 in Exercise 12.18, just look at the different sample incidence rates and make a personal judgment about which ones appear to be different from each other. Although such a procedure leaves something to be desired from a statistician's point of view, it is done quite a bit when it is "obvious" which incidence rates differ from each other. In the example of Table 12.4, where the sample incidence rates or proportions are 0.13, 0.20, and 0.30, it is "obvious" that the sample rates 0.13 and 0.30 are significantly different from each other. Whether 0.13 and 0.20 are significantly different, and whether 0.20 and 0.30 are significantly different, is not quite so obvious. Techniques to address this issue can be found in the references to this chapter under the topic of "partitioning of the χ^2 statistic."

As in the case for 2 × 2 tables, there are guidelines for larger contingency tables regarding how large the expected cell frequencies should be. One common guideline for tables larger than 2 × 2 is that no more than 20% of the expected cell frequencies be less than five *and* no expected frequency be less than one. Table 12.5 meets these conditions.

Exercise 12.19

You have now completed two χ^2 tests—one on a 2 × 2 table and one on a 2 × 3 table. This one statistical test of significance will be of immense use to you in your research and in understanding others' use (or misuse) of the test.

☐ What other common statistical tests of significance do you know of that are used in epidemiology?

Comment

There are many others tests of significance commonly used in epidemiology. For quantitative variables, t-tests and z-tests are often used, as well as analysis of variance and regression analysis. For nominal dependent variables, discriminant analysis sometimes is used. For ordinal variables, there are many nonparametric statistical techniques that can be used. We will leave exploration of these tests up to you.

Summary

The main points covered in this chapter include:

1. Variables can be classified as nominal, ordinal, or quantitative.

2. Quantitative variables are either discrete or continuous.

3. Arithmetic means can be calculated from quantitative data.

4. Proportions (rates) are applied to qualitative (categorical or nominal) data.

5. Watch out for researchers who may apply numbers to nominal or ordinal variables and then pretend that these variables are quantitative.

6. A commonly used statistical test of significance in epidemiology is the chi square test, which is used to test whether or not two nominal variables are associated.

7. Many other statistical tests of significance are available to deal with different combinations of nominal, ordinal, and quantitative variables.

References and Further Reading Sources

Topic	Reference number	Pages
Types of variables	1	65 79
	53	12–20
Chi square (χ^2) test	16	174–188
	29	152–179
	34	107–108
	46	73–80
	60	43–53
Partitioning of the χ^2 statistic	3	362–368
	60	51–53
Fisher's Exact Test	3	135–138
	60	54–57

Topic	Reference number	Pages
Other tests of significance	16	99–136
	29	133–151
	34	98–183
	53	173–241
	53	257–267
	60	24–42
	60	58–76

Associations and Their Meaning:
Are They Causal?

13

Previous chapters have dealt with various strategies and methods, potential errors and fallacies, tests of significance, and types of data and categories we use in epidemiology. These entities all come together when you consider the meaning of your findings and their possible implications. This chapter guides you in thinking through some of the ramifications of epidemiological inference in the search for causal factors.

Exercise 13.1

☐ In a study that compares the occurrence of a health attribute in two or more populations, what is the first consideration in seeing whether there is an association between the health attribute and the other characteristic (whether the null hypothesis is false)?

Write down your answer, then read the following discussion.

Comment

First, is there a numerical difference between the health indices (rates, means, and so forth) that describe the populations? More sophisticated techniques do exist to assess the presence of an association, such as correlation coefficients and other association coefficients, but we will not pursue them in this manual.

Exercise 13.2

☐ Assuming no numerical difference between the health indices for the various populatons, what considerations would you now have?

Comment

If you expected a difference, you might reflect upon potential errors in your method, sampling, data collection, and so forth, which may mask a true difference in the populations studied. If such errors are deemed likely to have happened, then the study needs to be redesigned and done again.

However, the absence of a numerical difference may be a reality, and that in itself may be very useful information. Two examples will illustrate this. First, certain populations in the world do not manifest the generally accepted association of increasing blood pressure with increasing age. Such absence of association may suggest a cultural or biological immunity to a disorder that afflicts the vast majority of older people in the world. Second, if you expected an improvement in health status among patients who received home visits and you did not observe this expected improvement, then it may be true that home visits do not improve health status. This finding of "no difference" is clearly of importance to health planners and administrators.

Another consideration, which you have learned about previously, can explain the absence of an expected difference in a study—a Type II error. That is, an association may truly exist in the population but, due to sampling variability, sample size, and the true differences in the parameters, the particular sample you use may not reflect the true differences in the population. Thus, in doing a statistical test of significance, you would not reject the null hypothesis (because there is no numerical difference) and you would be making a Type II error.

Exercise 13.3

☐ If there is a numerical difference, what is your next consideration?

Comment

We think the next consideration should be whether the difference is meaningful, or practically significant. Others, including you, may disagree with the particular order in which we deal with all these considerations; there is no established order.

By practical or meaningful difference, we mean a difference large enough to have important implications within the conceptual context of the study. For example, if a preventive program reduces the incidence of a rare nonfatal, mild disease by a small amount—say, 1 per 10,000—then this difference may not be meaningful in terms of continuing the preventive program, especially if it is expensive. Similarly, your study may show that a factor is independently associated with a disease with a relative risk slightly over 1, and this may be very important in the search for causes of the disease. However, the population attributable risk percent (PARP) may be quite small and, thus, not useful in terms of launching a program to reduce this factor.

The decision about the meaningfulness of a difference is yours, for you know the purpose of the study, its context, and the practicality of the findings. You will be helped in making your decision by reviewing published articles and by consulting with others who have made similar decisions.

Exercise 13.4

☐ If there is a numerical difference, and if it is meaningful, what explanations do you need to consider before accepting the association as nonartifactual?

Comment

You must consider at least five explanations, any or all of which may make your association artifactual (that is, spurious or secondary).

> 1. *Information bias.* You learned the relevance of this in Chapter 6, where we discussed potential hazards involved in labeling either disease states or characteristics.
>
> 2. *Selection bias.* In Chapter 8, we saw how selective forces can produce associations that are artifactual.
>
> 3. *Failure to control for confounding variables.* You first learned about this in Chapter 1 and subsequently throughout the manual. You will recall that knowledge about the factors already known to be associated with the occurrence of the health state or outcome (dependent variable, effect variable) is necessary to discern whether these factors are potential confounders in your study.
>
> 4. *Ecologic fallacy.* If ecologic indices are used in establishing the association, you know from Chapter 9 their potential in creating an artifactual association.
>
> 5. *Sampling variability or chance.* Using an appropriate statistical test of significance, which we discussed in Chapter 11, you can find out if the difference is likely to be due *only* to sampling variability (corresponding to a large p-value) or due to sampling variability *plus* true differences between the parameters (corresponding to a small p-value). A large p-value would lead you not to reject the null hypothesis, thus assuming that the difference is artifactual and produced only by sampling variability. A small p-value would lead you to reject the null hypothesis, thus assuming that the association really exists in the populaion.

Exercise 13.5

If your association "survives" the previous considerations about artifactuality and is meaningful, the association is likely to be real. Next it is necessary to determine whether the association is causal and where it fits into the network of causes.

☐ What evidence do you require in order to consider epidemiologic associations as causal?

Comment

This is probably the most difficult question in this manual
and the greatest challenge to epidemiological (or other behavioral) sciences. There are no absolutely correct answers to this question. We
offer you some rules of evidence to use when you consider whether an
association is causal. We hope that you will apply these rules, and any
other considerations, with scientific objectivity, despite your own or
others' subjective beliefs about the association.

The need for this objectivity was well stated by Marcus Aurelius many centuries ago: "If any man can convince and show me that
I do not think or act right, I will gladly change, for I seek truth, by
which no man was ever injured. But he is injured who abides in his
error and ignorance." (Aurelius M: *Meditations*. Roslyn, NY, Classics
Club, Walter J Black Inc, 1945)

The following rules of evidence are adapted from an article by Sir Austin Bradford Hill, which we urge you to read in full.[28] We present Hill's titles for his nine rules, but the explanations of them are paraphrased.

1. *Strength.* A large relative risk for a factor associated with a disease increases the likelihood that the association is causal. The size of the attributable risk bears no relation to this likelihood, but is of importance to the program implications of the association.

2. *Consistency.* If the association has been confirmed by others in different situations, in different populations, at different times, and with different methods of inquiry, then this increases the likelihood that the association is causal.

3. *Specificity.* If the association is particular to one factor and to one disease, this increases the likelihood that the association is causal. Such specificity is a rare event, because most diseases have more than one cause and suspected causes often are associated with more than one disease. As a result, Hill suggests that this rule of evidence not be overemphasized.

4. *Temporality.* Which came first, the disease or the characteristic? Obviously, in search of causality, we wish to show that the characteristic precedes the disease. Power is added to the inference that the association is causal if it is produced by a cohort or experimental study as opposed to a case-control or cross-sectional study.

5. *Biological gradient.* If the association demonstrates a dose-response relationship between the characteristic and the effect, then the association is more likely to be causal.

6. *Plausibility.* The association should be acceptable in the light of current biological knowledge. However, with the extremely rapid advance of this knowledge, the absence of such plausibility should not refute a causal inference.

7. *Coherence.* The association should be in accordance with other facts known about the disease, including its natural history.

8. *Experiment.* Associations derived from experiments—be they animal experiments, health programs, clinical traits, or natural experiments—add considerable weight to the evidence supporting a causal nature of the association.

9. *Analogy.* If similar associations have been shown to be causal, then, by analogy, the association is more likely to be causal. Because rubella in pregnancy is accepted as a cause of congenital abnormalities in infants, credence is added to the assertion of the causal nature of any new association of another infection or even a drug during pregnancy with congenital abnormalities.

Note: As you learned, and as Hill reminds us in his paper, statistical tests of significance do not contribute anything to the proof of causality in an association. Other references that will help you in addressing the issue of causality are listed at the end of this chapter.

It is salutary to complete this chapter with a quotation from Hill's paper on rules of evidence. "All scientific work is incomplete—whether it be observational or experimental. All scientific work is liable to be upset or modified by advancing knowledge. That does not confer upon us a freedom to ignore the knowledge we already have, or to postpone the action that it appears to demand at a given time. Who knows, asked Robert Browning, but the world may end tonight? True, but on available evidence most of us make ready to commute on the 8:30 next day."[28]

Summary

The main points covered in Chapter 13 include:

1. A series of considerations applied to associations to arrive at possible causality.

2. Exclusion of artifactuality by confounder.

3. Exclusion of bias and selection method pitfalls.

4. Measurement of sampling variability effect by statistical test of significance.

5. Possible causation considered using rules of evidence for moving toward such a decision.

6. No definite decision provided by any one study.

References and Further Reading Sources

Topic	Reference number	Pages
Causal inferences	1	162–169
about associations—	10	(article)
rules of evidence for	12	(article)
causality in	13	11–18
epidemiological	19	(article)
studies	27	173–195
	28	(article)
	29	312–323
	33	(article)
	36	289–321
	38	17–27
	40	94–111
	48	(article)
	51	(article)
	56	(article)
	59	(article)

Thinking Through a Study

14

In the previous chapters, we have considered many aspects of the epidemiological method. Now it is time to put all these aspects together and to consider how they are related in the course of a study.

Because epidemiology is an observational science that addresses the health of humans, many compromises between scientific rigor, practicality, and ethics have to be made in carrying out a study. Any researcher or investigator makes these compromises knowingly and takes them into account in interpreting the data and drawing conclusions from them. We can only touch upon some of the more important aspects of putting it all together and hope that you will address others as they arise in your pursuits.

As you can imagine, each time we seek answers about health status and disease, health behaviors, or health care there is a step-by-step process that can be followed beneficially. Some steps proceed sequentially and others go on concurrently. We present here a general outline of some of the factors that should be considered in carrying out a sound study. Like some pilots, one can hop in and take off, trusting to the mechanics and the winds to arrive at some desired destination. Or like other pilots, with whom we would prefer to ride, one can prepare the flight plan, check equipment lists, and consciously navigate throughout the flight. These processess all increase the probability of arriving safely at our correct destination, relying on logic and not serendipity.

Exercise 14.1

In the course of a conversation, the manager of a large manufacturing firm relates her concern to you. She believes, based on routine company statistics, that more cases of peptic ulcer are occurring

in the industry than in past years and that the increase is related some-
how to job dissatisfaction among workers. She suspects this may
explain a recent decline in worker productivity and a concomitant
decrease in company profits. If a study confirms her hunches, then she
intends to institute a program to improve satisfaction of the workers.
Because of your epidemiological skills, she enlists your help.

□ How would you begin?

Write down your answer, then read the discussion below.

Comment

Probably you would begin by asking to see the data that had
aroused her concern. These might include subjective or anecdotal histories of workers with ulcers and company statistics on sickness
absences or medical reimbursement claims. You might also want to
talk about the problem with a group of workers and other administrative people.

In addition, you would want a description of the total population of company workers in terms of as many social and demographic characteristics as available, such as sex, age, race, and so forth.
This will aid you in deciding whether you want to study the entire
work population in the company or just a portion of it. For example,
if a small percentage of the work force is male, you may wish to study
only females.

You will want also to confirm whether preemployment examinations identify applicants with an ulcer prior to employment, and
whether these applicants are excluded from employment. Because job
dissatisfaction at this company could not have caused an ulcer in these
persons, you will want to omit them from the population under study.

Exercise 14.2

☐ The manager shows you Table 14.1, which she prepared for the last board meeting. What do you conclude from this table?

Table 14.1   ***Employees Reported to Have an Ulcer, 1976–1980***

Year	Employees
1976	46
1977	123
1978	135
1979	124
1980	180

Comment

There is a secular increase in the number of workers reported to have an ulcer. But these are numerator (case) data and we need rates because the number of employees may have increased over the years. We recognize, too, that these data also may reflect increased *reporting* rather than an actual increase in the number of persons with an ulcer.

Exercise 14.3

☐ What data do you need now to further your explorations?

Comment

As we learned before, we need: (1) the number of employees, which would provide the PAR for each year, and (2) information about whether the numbers reported are for individual employees with ulcers or for episodes of ulcer problems. If they are the latter, the same employees may be counted more than once.

We realize that this apparent increase may be artifactual by virtue of bias, such as changes in diagnostic custom or in reporting or selective migration of workers with an ulcer in or out of the company. You can ask the manager if she has data or knowledge about these issues.

Exercise 14.4

With the data provided, you construct Table 14.2

Table 14.2   **Prevalence Rate per 100**
of Workers with an Ulcer, 1976–1980

Year	Rate
1976	2.3
1977	4.1
1978	5.4
1979	6.2
1980	10.0

□ Does this confirm the likelihood that there has been a secular increase in the prevalence rate?

Comment

We have a common base of comparison (per 100 workers), so the answer is "yes."

Exercise 14.5

The manager reiterates that she believes the problem is due to job dissatisfaction among workers and wants this hunch tested in a scientific manner.

☐ What is your next step?

Comment

You are now embarking on one of the most critical phases of a study, that of planning. The results of the entire effort can be no better than the preparation. This involves a lot of hard (and fun) work; it must be done before we start collecting data and feeding them into the computer.

The first step in planning is to outline the purpose of the study. At this stage, the aim is to make the study questions as specific as possible because it is more difficult, if not impossible, to answer unclear questions.

Studies need not be restricted to only one question; usually several questions are involved. Multiple working hypotheses are recommended to avoid overzealousness and attachment to one. While it is not necessary to limit a study to answering only one question, it is necessary, however, to limit the questions to a manageable number. Otherwise, with the study overburdened by too many questions and too many data, nothing will be answered well.

Exercise 14.6

Having confirmed the secular increase in the rate of workers with an ulcer, the task now is to state the question(s) or hypothesis(es) to be addressed by this study.

☐ a. How would you state simply the question of the association between dissatisfaction and occurrence of an ulcer?

☐ b. What other sorts of questions might you want to add?

☐ c. What would be your next step in planning the study?

Comment

a. Is there a positive association between job dissatisfaction and the occurrence of an ulcer? (If you want to state this in null hypothesis form, you can say: there is no association between job dissatisfaction and occurrence of an ulcer.)

b. You may be interested in whether this association is stronger among certain subgroups, for example among smokers as compared with nonsmokers or among those exposed to noisy working conditions as compared with those not exposed. These additional questions may come from your own conceptual framework and may not only enhance scientific knowledge, but may be important for the company if it goes ahead to implement a program to reduce job dissatisfaction among workers.

c. Despite your current knowledge, you actively search published material for guidance.

Exercise 14.7

☐ In what ways can published material help you in designing or planning a study?

.

Comment

1. A primary purpose is to find out what is really known about the topics under study. In this case, the topic is occurrence of ulcers, particularly in industrial populations. Few ideas come up that have not been addressed by others. Before you get too set on a charted course, it is important to know the experiences, options, findings, and methods of others who have given your study topic some attention. This information may be obtained from reading published material and by contacting investigators personally. Such personal contact can provide information beyond that included in publications, as well as information too recent to have been printed yet.

2. These pursuits may lead you into disciplines other than your own. In this particular study, you may need to read material from the areas of occupational medicine, epidemiology, industrial psychology, sociology, and so forth. Experts in these fields may be useful sources to contact. You will be careful, though, in applying the findings or methods from other studies to your population under study because populations studied by others will differ from your own. This does not mean that you do not use information from other studies, but simply that you do it with care.

3. The review of published material will help you identify potential confounding variables. You will have to account for these variables by (a) definition of study population, (b) method of sampling (if a sam-

ple is studied rather than the entire study population), or (c) analysis of data. In part, this identifies necessary information to be collected.

For example, you might find indications that type of work hazard exposure, level of responsibility, presence of a chronic disease, socioeconomic status, or length of employment are important to consider. The number of variables that must be considered as potentially confounding is usually a function of how much research has been done on the subject, that is, how many associations have already been discovered to be potential confounders in your study. You will remember that potential confounders must be associated with the exposure variable (dissatisfaction) and with the effect or outcome (occurrence of an ulcer).

4. You may benefit by examining the research designs others have used in answering similar questions, not only what designs were used but what were the strengths and weaknesses they attributed in interpreting the findings.

5. You may learn from your review what rates of occurrence of job dissatisfaction and ulcers are reported, especially in similar occupational settings. These will guide you in estimating the number of reported ulcer cases and of dissatisfied workers, and will also help in determining the size of the sample(s) you may wish to use in your study.

6. The review may provide an indication of the various statistical and other analytical techniques that other workers have used in dealing with a similar problem.

7. The review may provide the various indices and instruments others have used to measure your variables, including their reliability and validity as used in those studies. These may include criteria for ascertaining and diagnosing ulcers and ways of measuring worker satisfaction. By providing information about the utility of these instruments, such reports may give you more confidence about using the instruments in your study. It is a waste of effort to invent a new measuring instrument if a valid, reliable, and suitable one is available. In addition, use of similar instruments or indices enables you to compare the findings of your study with those of other investigators.

8. The review will provide names of others working on similar problems whom you could contact for further information.

A note of advice: As you do your review of published information, elaborate on the conceptual framework addressing your study, and develop your ideas on methods of ascertaining cases of ulcers, measuring satisfaction, analyzing your findings, and so forth, *do write them down*. However good your memory is, make sure to record the bases of your decisions for your study, the reasons for compromises that you make, the reasons you chose one method or another. All these issues and more will arise as you read relevant publications and discuss your study with others; not to record them invites later regret. After the study is done, you will want to include your considerations and justifications in any report you write or present, and only on-going recording of the development of your considerations and decisions will allow rational explanation of them later. There is no perfect study, but one needs to make compromises knowingly and substantiate the choices.

For many of us, scientific writing is not easy; for all of us, it is essential.

Exercise 14.8

□ In considering choice of study design, you may prefer to do a cohort or historical cohort study. Are these options feasible?

Comment

The prevalence rate of ulcer in this firm has ranged from 2.3 to 10.0 per 100 during 1976–1980. The incidence rate is almost certainly less than this, although the data presented so far give no indication of what the incidence rate may be. Although you may wish to do a cohort study, the possibility of a fairly low incidence rate and a relatively small population of workers will discourage your choice of this option. Further, you know that a cohort study will take a fairly long period of time; can the manager wait that long for an answer? No, she cannot.

Perhaps they have good data so you can carry out an historical cohort study. The manager does have past data on job dissatisfaction in the form of complaints, nonsickness absences, and poor relationships with other workers. But with the small anticipated incidence rate for an ulcer from other studies and the small population at risk in this study, an historical cohort study is not feasible.

Exercise 14.9

You rapidly discard any notions of an experimental study; such would be unethical and inhumane in this situation because it would involve manipulating job dissatisfaction among workers and then assessing the effect upon incidence of an ulcer.

☐ Now, what study designs are left for you to consider?

Comment

Your learning suggests two other possibilities:

1. One is a cross-sectional study in which you will associate job dissatisfaction with the concurrent presence of an ulcer at one point in time. However, you will recall that this does not allow one to establish any time relationship between job dissatisfaction and the occurrence of an ulcer, that is, to establish which one happened first.

2. Another possibility is a case-control study, in which you will compare the job dissatisfaction histories of workers with an ulcer (the cases) with similar histories of workers without an ulcer (controls).

As compared with a cross-sectional study, a case-control study is indicated when the condition (ulcer) is rare or when you are looking for a time relationship between the presumed cause and effect. In addition, it will quantify the relative risk and, under certain assumptions, permit you to estimate the etiologic fraction, the population attributable risk percent that would give the industry a reasonable estimate of the number of cases of ulcer that would be preventable if job dissatisfaction can be removed.

Hence, under these circumstances, you would choose a case-control study.

Exercise 14.10

□ Pursuing a case-control study, how would you identify workers with an ulcer (cases)?

Comment

Well, the best method is a clinical examination of all workers, but that may not be feasible or even ethical or even to the liking of the workers. In your readings, you would probably come across an instrument used by other investigators to measure the presence of an ulcer. It consists of four to five questions about symptoms that suggest the presence of an ulcer. This instrument seems eminently cheaper, quicker, and a reasonably satisfactory way of identifying cases.

Exercise 14.11

□ What else would you want to know about this instrument before deciding to use it?

Comment

The use of instruments available from other studies is a commonly addressed issue in epidemiology. Generally, if possible, we would like to repeat the tests of reliability and validity of the instrument in our own study population or one similar to it, especially if the instrument was devised in another cultural setting. To check validity, as you remember, you apply the instrument to known ulcer cases, perhaps obtained from clinical settings, and to non-ulcer cases. For reproducibility or reliability, you would have to apply the same instrument on more than one occasion to a number of persons. If the sensitivity, specificity, and reliability of the instrument are high enough, you may elect to use it.

Just as there is no perfect study, there is no perfect instrument or set of diagnostic criteria to determine a case. One uses these instruments or diagnostic criteria because they are the best available, knowing that there are possible errors in so doing.

Exercise 14.12

☐ On behalf of the company, the manager accepts the proposed case-control study. What is the first step now in implementing your study?

Comment

Draw up an initial study protocol, including the definition of the study population, which variables you need to collect, how they should be collected, how they should be coded, how cases and controls will be identified, any matching of cases and controls that is to be done, and any other relevant details you can think of. Consultation may be needed at this stage with various experts unless you have the skills yourself or already have used consultants at an earlier stage.

At this stage, you should ask a series of questions about each piece of information to be gathered. Such questions would include, among others: (1) Why is this information being gathered? (2) Is the variable to be used in the identification of cases and controls? (3) Is it a variable to be used in measuring the presumed cause (job dissatisfaction)? (4) Is it a potential confounding variable? (5) Is it to be used for administrative purposes only? (6) Beyond that, is it ethical to ask people for that information? (7) How does this variable fit into the analytical scheme for this study?

Any variable or piece of information that is not important to answer the hypotheses or questions raised or for administration of the study should not be collected. All too often, studies are carried out that one might describe as shotgun epidemiology: a bunch of data is collected and shoved through the computer; some findings come out and establish an answer in need of a question. Do not collect data "because they may show something" or "because you may want them later." Collect what you need to answer your study questions and nothing more.

Exercise 14.13

☐ Let us take an example of this. Would you obtain the name, age, sex, race, and address of all cases and all controls? If so, why?

Comment

Names can only have relevance for administrative purposes, for example, to check the medical history or for identification of the workers in the company. However, if names beginning with a particular letter or five-letter names have been shown to be associated with job dissatisfaction and the presence of an ulcer, then names would be collected and dealt with as a potentially confounding variable. This event is unlikely, given the current state of knowledge.

Age almost invariably is collected because it is associated with almost all health outcomes and factors associated with these outcomes. You will recall in previous exercises that we referred to this as a universal variable (effect modifier). In your review of the published material, you probably would find that the presence of an ulcer is related to age and, further, age (perhaps) may be associated with job dissatisfaction. Hence, age is a potential confounder in your study, as well as in most epidemiological studies. Of course, you will confirm its confounding nature in your study when you analyze your data.

A similar argument is possible for the collection of data on sex and race. Address often is used for administrative purposes in checking identity of the worker or to relocate subjects if followup data will be collected. Sometimes address is used as one indicator of socioeconomic status.

Each and every variable *must* have a reason; if in doubt, leave it out.

Exercise 14.14

☐ Your lurking concerns about the sample you will use confront you vividly when the manager asks how many workers you need to study. What considerations do you have in replying to this question?

Comment

The size of the sample to be used in this study, and in many studies, is always a difficult problem because the cost, feasibility, and other factors often demand compromising the ideal sample size. There is no easy answer to the manager's question.

The first thing to determine is the number of cases you would like to have in your study. As you learned before, this is influenced by the difference in job dissatisfaction between the two groups that the manager considers meaningful, or, alternatively, the magnitude of the relative risk that is meaningful to the manager. It is also influenced by what levels of α and β you recommend. Further, sample size will depend upon the range of scores on job dissatisfaction you expect to obtain. Also included in these deliberations is whether you will use an equal number of cases and controls or two, three, four, or more controls per case. If matching of cases and controls is your procedure of choice to deal with some confounding variables, then multiple controls per case (perhaps up to four) is often recommended, but it is not that easy in practice to find multiple controls that match given cases. Hence, especially when matching cases with controls, you may need to settle for fewer than the ideal number of controls per case. In fact, many case-control studies are done with an equal number of controls as cases. Consultation may be of use here in helping you decide on the number of cases and controls you would like to have.

Having determined the desired number of cases for the study, it is easy from known rates of occurrence of ulcer to determine how many workers need to be examined to obtain the desired number of cases and controls. For example, if 80 cases are needed and the rate of ulcer is 20 per 1,000, then you need to examine about 4,000 workers in order to obtain the 80 cases. Obviously, you would have identified 3,920 controls from which you could select the controls for your study. All too often this is not possible, either because the company is not that big or the process is too time consuming or too expensive. Once again, you may need to compromise and settle for fewer cases than desired.

Exercise 14.15

☐ The sample that you determine as necessary for the study is too large to be feasible, according to the manager. What do you do now?

Comment

First, explain that this sample size was necessary for all the specifications made by you and the manager. If the sample size is not feasible, then either compromise on some of the specifications or carry out the study on the largest possible sample size. By using acceptable sampling procedures, make sure that the sample is as representative of the study population as possible. *Do the study*, knowing that your compromise of a smaller sample size will reduce the chances of statistical significance at your preset levels, that is, increase Type II error (β).

All too frequently, we are confronted by logistic, financial, and situational realities and do studies on available or convenience samples. But we do this knowingly, and are then simply more circumspect about the conclusions we draw from that sample.

Exercise 14.16

☐ You have revised the protocol, including the sampling plan for selection of cases and controls. You show it to the manager and representatives of the workers. Do you need to do a pretest?

Comment

Yes, generally speaking. The pretest of a study protocol will provide you with considerable help in the ultimate study. What you are aiming to do with your pretest is to carry out the study, as if it were real, on a sample as similar to your study population as is possible. It is not advisable to carry out the pretest on a sample of the actual workers who will be in the study but rather attempt to obtain a sample of workers from another similar industry. The pretest will indicate the understandability of the questions, the ease and comfort of the persons being questioned, the time duration for each interview, and the number of interviews that can be done in any one day. On that basis, the number of staff required to carry out the study can be estimated. The experience of the pretest will suggest training needs and any changes that may be required in the final version of the protocol. A pretest can confirm for you the expected number of cases in the study population and the distribution of variables that you could expect in your study population.

If your pretest sample is large enough, you conceivably may be able to decide upon categories for your variables, if you wish to categorize some of them. You may well be able to test your analytic models on your pretest data to see the extent to which the data meet the assumptions of the planned statistical tests.

In some studies, a pretest is not carried out; but when feasible, it is advisable.

Exercise 14.17

☐ The pretest has been completed. What do you do now, prior to carrying out the actual study?

Comment

Modify the protocol in the light of the administrative and substantive findings of your pretest. Of course, the protocol will include an approved, informed consent form to be signed by all participants in the study. Obtain approval of the revised protocol from the manager, representatives of the workers, and all consultants. Staff will need to be recruited and staff training will be instituted.

Exercise 14.18

☐ Are there any more preparatory steps prior to implementing the actual study?

Comment

No. Go ahead with the first stage of the study, collecting information to identify cases and controls (noncases). You will be collecting these data on the entire study population if it is small and does not contain very many cases or on a random sample from the study population if it is large and contains many more cases than you need for your study.

Ensure throughout that the interviewers who administer questionnaires or who carry out any required examinations have been trained to, and continue to, apply the protocol in a consistent, objective manner. As the data are received, they should be scrutinized for errors, omissions, and possible biases in terms of the interviewers.

Exercise 14.19

□ The data have been collected and are in hand. What is the next step in the identification of cases and controls?

Comment

Code the data. Apply your pretest criteria for a case (a person with an ulcer). This gives you a listing of cases for your study. The controls are chosen from the list of noncases.

Exercise 14.20

☐ Now you may want to consider matching cases and controls on some variables. How would you proceed in doing this matching?

Comment

In most studies, investigators decide on what variables they will match, based on review of other studies. Many times they match on the universals such as age, sex, and race, in addition to particular variables relevant to the outcome and antecedent under study. If you used this procedure, you would now match your cases to controls, whether you choose one, two, three or four controls per case.

Recently the following alternative approach has been suggested. Given the cases and controls you have identified, and *also* assuming that you have measured the antecedent variable on these subjects, use these data to identify which variables are confounding variables *in your data at hand*. Once confounding variables are identified in your study, you may wish to match in order to control on some or all of these confounding variables. In this approach, the variables to be matched on are *not* decided upon before collecting the data but *after* the data are collected This procedure may not be feasible if it is very expensive to collect information on the antecedent variable.

You will recall the following attributes of a confounding variable. First, it should not be part of the causative network because if it is, we want to quantify its association with the outcome variable. If you make the cases and controls similar on this variable by matching, then you will not be able to measure the strength of the association between cause and outcome. Second, the association between the confounding variable and the outcome variable should be predictive; that is, the confounding variable must precede the outcome variable. Third, the confounding variable or the associations found cannot confound if they are not found *in your data*. Fourth, the confounding variable should be shown to be associated with the outcome variable in the unexposed group; it should change the outcome (effect) measure without the exposure variable.

Exercise 14.21

☐ If you cannot find the ideal number of controls for each case, what then?

Comment

Obtain and use as many controls per case as you can. Sometimes it is advised to have the *same* number of controls per case so that the statistical analysis does not become unduly complicated.

Exercise 14.22

☐ What is the first thing you will look for in the data?

Comment

If you matched controls with cases, compare the matching characteristics of the cases and their controls to assess the success in matching. Clearly you need to see that the two groups are similar on matched criteria. It may be of interest to compare cases and controls on a variable that was not matched, for example, a variable that is not relevant to the study. If this "dummy" variable is similarly distributed among cases and controls, chances are good you have done well in matching.

Be warned against using only the median or mean in making these comparisons because, alone, they are not good indicators of whether the characteristic has the same distribution in both groups. For example, the distribution of age can be quite different in two groups but yet the mean age of each group can be the same. You learned all this before.

Exercise 14.23

□ You find matching was good, and no important or significant differences were found between cases and controls on these matched variables. What is the next step in looking at the data?

Comment

Look for further confounding variables among variables on which you have not matched. If you find no further confounding variables, proceed to the test of your hypothesis. If you do find further confounding variables, then suitable adjustment by a control table or other statistical techniques of adjustment will be necessary in order to test your hypothesis. We cannot elaborate on these methods here, but they include stratification of confounder scores, regression techniques, and others. If you are uncertain, seek guidance from references on the subject or from persons who know how.

Exercise 14.24

□ Can you, at last, test your hypothesis?

Comment

Yes. You have confirmed good matching on the cases and controls and identified other variables that will need to be adjusted for since they are confounders. Now, answer the initial question by calculating relative risk (risk ratios) for dissatisfied workers.

If there are no further confounding variables to be controlled on in the analysis, this would be done as in Chapter 3 on case-control studies.

Exercise 14.25

□ Assume that you find the risk for ulcers among dissatisfied workers to be 3.7 times that of satisfied workers, that is, the relative risk is 3.7. Further, this is statistically significant at your preset value of Type I error (or α). What is the next step?

Comment

Present it to the manager, both orally and in a full written report. This is the most difficult, perhaps, of all tasks, for all too many of us have great difficulty communicating our thoughts, impressions, and interpretations. However, one owes this to the company and, in a general sense, to the scientific world, for however small and however humble the study may be, it may well contribute to the advancement of knowledge about that particular topic.

The writing of the report should be done as succinctly and scientifically as possible, with conclusions made in the light of the findings and not one's impressions. The whole field of epidemiology is one of relative uncertainty because of its observational nature, so all conclusions may be guarded, but some conclusions should be drawn. The conclusions you draw from the study must encompass the compromises you made and other related problems that arose in the study. Such honestly presented ultimate explanations of your findings are expected of scientists, for they indicate that you are aware of them, have no interest other than a scientific one in reaching conclusions, and ultimately recognize that there is no perfect study.

Exercise 14.26

☐ The manager accepts the report (pays your fee, it is hoped) and asks your opinion about what needs to be done. What further suggestions do you have?

Comment

First, you calculate the population attributable risk from the risk ratio and inform her what reduction of ulcers is to be anticipated, theoretically, if dissatisfaction can be removed, with no other ill effects. This is based on your confirmation of her hunch of the association between job dissatisfaction and presence of ulcer. However, before recommending a company-wide program to remove or reduce dissatisfaction, you should recommend an experiment to confirm whether dissatisfaction *can* be removed or reduced, followed by the anticipated effect of reduction in ulcers. Such an experiment, you will recall, is a randomized clinical trial.

Exercise 14.27

☐ If the randomized clinical trial proves to be effective in removing dissatisfaction with the consequent reduction of ulcers, what would you then recommend to the company?

Comment

Recommend that the intervention (treatment) for removal of dissatisfaction be implemented for the whole company, with monitoring over subsequent years to confirm the anticipated reduction in ulcer occurrence.

Also, finish your report, and publish it, for you have done a first-rate (but never perfect) scientific investigation of an epidemiological problem.

Addendum

We have used a case-control strategy as an example, in putting it all together. Similar steps and considerations would apply to cross-sectional, cohort, or experimental studies. In all of these, you would pose the specific questions; seek help from published material and other researchers; estimate the necessary sample size, given specifications; test for reliability and validity; do a pretest; redesign your protocol based on pretest results; conduct the study; analyze the data; reach conclusions; and produce a written report.

This chapter leaves much unaddressed; some excellent references are listed with it. But in the end, doing the study to the best of your knowledge and ability and the experience of doing it (and making errors) are your best guide to progressive learning.

Summary

Chapter 14 outlines the main considerations in carrying out a study:

1. There is no perfect study.

2. The progressive steps in addressing a problem or question are sequential and concurrent.

3. A review of published material and opinions of other researchers will help.

4. The statement of the problem, question, or hypothesis is based upon specifications that include what a meaningful difference or degree of association is as well as statistical inferential requirements.

5. Compromises in the size of the sample to be studied, based upon the previous specifications, are likely.

6. A study protocol is drawn up.

7. Tests of reliability and validity should be carried out, where indicated.

8. If possible, the protocol is pretested, which provides information regarding the administrative cost and feasibility of the method.

9. The protocol is modified, based upon pretest results.

10. The study is carried out according to the modified protocol.

11. The data are analyzed, confounding variables are considered and controlled, and then the hypothesis is tested or the question is answered.

12. Conclusions and recommendations are drawn, however tentative they may be.

13. The study is described in written form, including the reasons for the compromises made and their implications for the conclusions. A written report is necessary so that interested persons can learn from your study.

References and Further Reading Sources

Topic	Reference number	Pages
Thinking through and doing a study	1	13–38
	1	170–175
	27	196–215
	29	40–50
	30	359–383
	34	2–15
General books on epidemiology	4	
	5	
	6	
	24	
	25	
	26	
	27	
	31	
	36	
	38	
	40	
	45	
	46	
	47	
	61	
	67	

Glossary

Brief definitions are given for the major terms used in this manual. Further explanation and examples can be found by referring to the pages listed. The **boldface** page numbers indicate where the term is first introduced or where it is best explained.

Adjusted rate.   A rate that has been statistically adjusted to "remove" any effects a given variable may have in relation to the comparisons being made.   **12**, 18, 19, 20, 21, 22, 23, 26, 27, 185

Age-specific rate.   The rate of an outcome calculated for a certain age group. Only people in the designated age brackets are included in the numerator and denominator.   **9**, 10, 16, 17, 18, 26, 27, 28

Alpha (α).   The probability of rejecting a null hypothesis when it is true (Type I error).   55, **232**, 234

Alternate hypothesis.   A statistical statement that expresses a relationship between two (or more) variables.   **226**

Artifactual.   See Spurious.   **43**

Association.   As one variable changes, there is a concomitant or resultant change in the quantity or quality of another variable.   **41**, 43, 44, 63, 73, 74, 80, 81, 91, 123, 185, 239, 265

At risk.   Capable of experiencing the health state under study.   **3**, 93, 96, 114

Attributable risk.   A figure that quantifies the amount of risk due to a certain characteristic. It is obtained by subtracting the incidence rate for the group without the characteristic from the rate for the group with the characteristic.   **107**, 109, 111, 220

Berkson's fallacy.   Nonrepresentativeness of cases because those cases who seek care are selectively different from those who do not.   **86**, 89

Beta (β).   The probability of not rejecting a null hypothesis when it is false (Type II error).   55, **233**, 234

Bias.   A conscious or unconscious tendency to mislabel observations in a nonrandom (systematic) manner.   116, 147, **148**

Bimodal distribution.   A frequency distribution with two peaks (modes).   **212**

Biological variability.   The differences in assessment or test results due to the natural changeability of individual subjects over time.   **159**

Biostatistics.   The mathematical science of quantifying observed phenomena to describe and analyze epidemiological comparisons.   **viii**, 217

Case-control method.   A method of study that can support and test hypotheses about supposed causes. The data collection is retrospective, that is, the past characteristics and events are analyzed for cases and noncases.   **67**, 78, 79, 89

Case (incident) control method.   A case-control study where only new cases are studied or the time of manifestation of the effect is known—for example, from clinical records. This avoids selective survival.   **79**, 82

Case fatality ratio.   The death rate of cases; deaths of cases are the numerator and total cases are the denominator.   **44**, 104, 120, 121, 122

Case follow-up study.   The descriptive epidemiology of the natural history of diseases, including recuperation.   142, **143**, 146

Case-series study.   A study of cases only, with no control group for comparison.   **70**, 87

Categorical variable.   A variable created by collapsing a larger number of values into a few categories, or one that by its nature is not suited to a long continuum of possible values.   177, 178, **240**

Causal.   Inferring from findings that an antecedent leads to the health state under study.   49, **50**, 53, 68, 69, 80, 270, 271, 272, 295

Chi square (χ^2) test.   A statistical test applied to nominal or categorical data.   **244**, 248, 251, 252, 262

Clinical epidemiology.   The application of the science of epidemiology and biostatistics to clinical practice.

Clinical hunch   An idea that arises during clinical care that can be a valuable source of epidemiological hypotheses.   **30**, 32, 69, 70, 71, 87, 145

Clinical trial.   An experimental study to test the efficacy and potential side effects of an intervention such as a drug, vaccine, or medical device.   **132**, 134, 136, 137, 138, 146, 300

Cohort.   A group of persons who have characteristics in common and are studied prospectively.   **92**

Cohort effect.   A special age group going through life with a high or low rate of a condition and carrying this characteristic with them into successive age categories over time.   **45**, 207, 216

Cohort study.   A study design that looks forward in time from baseline data. Health status and related characteristics are assessed and later reassessed to determine which characteristics preceded or caused newly developed health outcomes. This design best allows for estimates of the probability or risk of developing the outcome. **69**, 91

Confounding variable. A variable related to a health state that is distributed differently in different groups causing confusion (introduces artifactual estimates of effect) in comparing the rates of health states in the groups. **12**, 13, 14, 28, 43, 45, 221, 269, 282, 295, 297

Continuous variable. A quantitative variable that can have an unlimited number of values on a measurable continuum. **243**

Control group. Used in case-control or experimental study designs as a comparison for testing hypotheses. 68, 71, **72**, 78, 87, 89, 134, 135, 138, 139

Control table. Presentation of data relating two or more variables while showing or controlling for the effect of other variables. **18**, 19

Controlling for. Examining the effect of one variable on the health outcome while taking into account the effect of another; for example, looking at death rates by sex within specific age groups. **15**, 18, 19

Cross-sectional method. A study design that shows concurrently existing characteristics and health outcomes. Like a picture of the situation at a specific time, it cannot answer questions about cause and effect or whether the characteristics preceded the outcome. **29**, 37, 56, 57, 65, 94

Crude rate. The rate of an outcome calculated without any restrictions (such as age, race, or sex) on who is counted in the numerator or denominator. **5**, 11

Cumulative incidence (rate). An incidence rate that covers a specified time period—for example, one year or five years—and for which all subjects are followed over the same period of time. **95**

Death registration states. States registering deaths in a uniform manner and contributing to the national vital statistics system. **2**

Degrees of freedom (df). For chi-square tests, the number of cells in the table whose expected number of subjects does not depend upon the expected number of subjects in other cells. **251**, 253, 254

Dependent variable. Usually the health outcome under study where the aim is to determine to what extent it is dependent on or a result of other variables. **49**, 243, 244

Descriptive epidemiology. Describing the frequency and relative distributions of health and disease in populations.

Direct method of age adjustment. Uses a standard population and applies the age-specific rates of the populations being compared to determine the expected number of events in the standard population. 22, **23**

Discrete variable. A quantitative variable that can assume only a limited set of values no matter how precise measurement techniques are. **243**

Dose-response relationship. As the amount of exposure to a risk factor increases, the rate of the effect of exposure increases. **123**, 124, 271

Ecologic fallacy.   An error in interpreting associations between ecologic indices. It is committed by mistakenly assuming that, because the majority of a group has a characteristic, the characteristic is related to a health state common in the group.   **195**, 198, 269

Ecologic index.   A system of classification that applies the majority characteristic of an entire group to all individuals within the group, irrespective of individual characteristics.   195, 198, 200, **204**

Effect modifier.   A variable that modifies or influences the effect (for instance, disease, outcome). It is often part of the causative network, in an interactive sense.   **14**, 15, 28, 289

Epidemic.   The occurrence of a higher rate of a health state than would be expected, based on past experience.

Epidemiology.   A science concerned with the distribution of the occurrence of health, disease, and health behavior in human populations. It is both a body of knowledge and a method.   **vii**

Etiologic fraction.   See population attributable risk percent.   **108**

Exhaustive categories.   All subjects are classifiable in some category of the classification scheme for the variable.   **180**

Experimental epidemiology.   Introducing a suspected cause and measuring the subsequent effect in populations. Usually used to evaluate the efficacy of some intervention procedure.   **69**, 131

Extrapolation.   Making numerical predictions for the future based on past and current rates or quantities.   **5**

False negatives.   In tests of validity, labeling cases or the presence of a characteristic incorrectly, that is, categorizing cases as noncases or failing to identify the characteristic when in fact it was present.   **161**, 163

False positives.   In tests of validity, labeling noncases or the absence of a characteristic incorrectly, that is, categorizing noncases as cases or identifying a characteristic when in fact it was not present.   **161**, 163

Fisher's Exact Test for 2 × 2 tables.   A statistical test of significance that can be used in place of a chi square test when the expected number of subjects in some cells is less than five.   **257**

Flow diagram.   A diagram that shows the progressive divisions of the original population into the groups from which inferences flow.   96, 98, 103, **137**, 142

Historical cohort study.   A cohort study done on a cohort defined in the past.   **127**

Hybrid study.   A combination of the case-incident-control method and cohort method in one study.   **118**

Incidence.   The occurrence of new cases during a specified period of time.   **95**, 94, 219

Incidence density (rate).   A rate where the numerator is person-years, for example, rather than persons, because all subjects have *not* been followed for the same period of time.   **95**

Incidence study. *See* Cohort study. **69**, 91

Independent association. A relationship between two variables that holds when controlling or adjusting for other variables. **63**, 64

Independent variable. A characteristic or situation being considered for its relation (possibly causative) to a health outcome. **49**, 243, 244

Indirect association. A dependent relationship between two variables, which appears to exist only because of the confounding influence of a third variable and disappears when the third variable is controlled. Secondary association. **53**, 269

Indirect method of age adjustment. Standard rates are applied to the populations being compared in order to calculate the expected number of events, which is then compared with the observed number of events. **23**, 24

Information bias. *See* Bias. **148**

Interobserver reliability. The degree to which two (or more) different observers classify consistently among themselves observations on a group of subjects. **148**, 155, 156

Intra-observer reliability. The degree to which one observer classifies observations the same at two different points in time. **148**, 152, 153, 154

Life-table analysis. A method of including people in a cohort study for different durations during the overall study period. **114**

Linear relationship. When two variables are considered together, the first increases as the second increases (or decreases), so that, when plotted graphically, a straight line results. **9**

Matching. A technique for controlling on variables that are actual or potential confounders. **75**, 89, 140, 295, 296, 297

Mortality rate (death rate). The probability of dying within a specified time period, multiplied by a constant. **4**, 3, 5, 15, 16

Mutually exclusive categories. Each subject appears in only one category. **180**

Natural history of disease. The description of what happens following the development of disease, including complications, cure, death, symptom change, remissions, and so forth. Systematic prospective study can quantify the probability of these events for a group of cases. 142, **143**, 146

Negative (inverse) association. As the amount of the characteristic increases, the rate of the health state decreases.

Nominal variable. The data from these variables name things; they do not measure or quantify amounts. Also called qualitative variables. 177, **240**

Nonparametric statistics. Statistical techniques that can be used on nominal or ordinal data. **261**

Null hypothesis. A statement expressing no relationship between two (or more) variables or no difference. **225**, 226, 227

Odds ratio. A technique for estimating relative risk from case-control studies. *See* Relative odds ratio. 83, **84**, 109

Ordinal variable.   A variable having values that can be meaningfully ordered or ranked, for example, from less to more, from small to large. **242**

Parameter.   The true value of a population is health attribute. **54**

Parametric statistics.   Statistical techniques that can be used on quantitative data. **261**

Period prevalence.   The number or rate of individuals with a specific health outcome at the time period when the count is made. **37**

Placebo.   A nontreatment or pseudo-teatment used in an experimental study which is believed to be effective by the subject. **135**, 136, 146

Point prevalence study.   *See* Cross-sectional method. **37**

Population at risk (PAR).   Those individuals capable of developing a specified health state; they become the denominator for calculating the rate of the health state. **3**, 5, 6, 94, 98, 183, 278

Population attributable risk percent (PARP).   A measure of the benefit derived by modifying a risk factor. **107**, 108, 109, 111, 219, 220

Positive association.   As the amount of the characteristic increases, the rate of the health state increases. **43**, 281

Practical significance.   Exists if the findings have important implications within the conceptual context of the study. **267**, 268

Prevalence.   The number or rate of cases that exist (prevail) at a specified time. **34**, 35, 36, 39, 46, 48, 61, 96

Probability.   An estimate of the frequency or likelihood of the occurrence of an event. 4, **5**

Prospective study.   *See* Cohort study. **69**, 91

P-value.   The probability of obtaining a difference between sample estimates as large as the observed difference, given that the null hypothesis is true. 229, **228**, 235, 236

Qualitative variables.   Can be named or classified but not quantified as to "how much." Also called nominal variables. **240**

Quantitative variables.   Can be measured in terms of "how much." 177, 178, **240**

Quasi-experimental.   Research designs in which the investigator does not have as much control as in an experimental design. **133**

Randomization.   Assigning people to treatment and control groups in an unbiased manner so as to produce groups similar on characteristics not controlled by other methods. Sometimes, called random assignment of subjects to groups or random allocation. **139**, 140, 146

Randomized clinical trial.   A clinical trial in which subjects have been randomly assigned to the various groups in the study. **140**

Rate.   A numerical statement of the frequency of an event obtained by dividing the number of individuals experiencing the event (the numerator) by the total number capable of experiencing the event (the denominator or the population at risk) and multiplying by a constant such as 100 or 1,000.   **1,** 28, 33, 34, 58, 59, 60, 175

Relationship.   *See Association.*   **41**

Relative odds (or odds ratio).   Percentage of cases that were exposed to the presumed antecedent divided by the percentage of controls that were similarly exposed. It is used sometimes in case-control studies as an estimate of relative risk.   **84,** 89

Relative risk.   A ratio obtained by dividing the incidence rate of one group by the incidence rate of another group. If the rates were equal, the resulting relative risk would be one.   82, **103,** 105, 109, 110, 125, 219, 271

Reliability (reproducibility).   The degree to which observations are repeatedly classified the same.   147, **148,** 159, 160, 171, 172, 187, 287

Reproducibility.   *See Reliability.*   **148**

Retrospective.   Looking back. Retrospective study means case-control study.   **68**

Risk.   The probability or likelihood of a health-related event or outcome.   **143**

Risk factor.   A characteristic, behavior, or experience that increases the probability of developing (causes) a negative health status.   143, **225**

Sample.   A group of subjects selected for study from a larger population or universe.   **32,** 55, 65, 102

Sample size.   The number of subjects chosen for study to represent a larger population.   86, 267, **290,** 291

Sampling variability.   The differences between findings for all possible samples from the same or equivalent populations. It is possible to draw many different samples from any one population, and each one would provide somewhat different findings.   **54,** 55, 102, 217, 221, 222, 223, 224, 227, 228, 267, 269

Secondary association.   Associations produced by confounding variables. *See Indirect association.*   **53,** 269

Secular trend.   Refers to the trend over time.   91, **95,** 277

Selection.   Factors that affect the composition of the populations studied so as to confuse comparisons between groups, that is, produce artifactual findings.   116, **183,** 188, 192, 193

Selective survival.   The result of differences between those who die and those who live; those who survive can have characteristics related to maintaining life that confound retrospective studies of the health outcome causing mortality.   **45,** 79, 86

Sensitivity.   In tests of validity, the percent of all true cases identified correctly.   **162,** 163, 164, 168, 170

Simple attributable risk.   *See Attributable risk.*   **107**

Specificity.   In tests of validity, the percent of all true noncases identified correctly.   **162,** 163, 164, 168, 170

Spurious (artifactual).   When applied to associations, it means they are not real but rather false relationships produced by methodological errors or confounding variables.   **43**, 221, 269

Standardized Mortality Ratio (SMR).   The ratio of observed events to events expected if standard rates are applied to the study populations. It is usually the figure used in indirect adjustments.   **24**, 25, 27

Standard population.   An arbitrary distribution of a characteristic (for example, age) is used as a common standard for two groups when comparing their rates.   **19**, 21

Statistical tests of significance.   Methods of determining the likelihood that estimates of population parameters are different due to sampling variability only.   102, **217**, 267

Tables.   A way to present and summarize numerical data in an organized fashion.   **1**, 8

True negatives.   In tests of validity, labeling noncases or the absence of characteristics correctly.   **161**, 163

True positives.   In tests of validity, labeling cases or characteristics correctly.   **161**, 163

Type I error.   Rejection of a null hypothesis that is really true. *See* Alpha.   55, **230**, 231, 234

Type II error.   Failure to reject a null hypothesis that is really false. *See* Beta.   55, **230**, 231, 234

Universal variables (effect modifiers).   Characteristics that in nature generally modify many health events and need to be considered when comparing groups.   **14**, 15, 239, 289

Unweighted average.   Gives an equal weight to each component of the average.   **199**

Validity.   The correctness of labeling; the ability of a criterion or tool to measure what it claims to measure, or the correctness of participants' reports.   147, **160**, 161, 172, 187, 188, 287

Weighted average.   Gives different weights to each component of the average.   **199**

References

These references are numbered for referral purposes throughout this manual. They include not only those used in this manual but also other available references. The list, of course, is not exhaustive. Peruse and use them before buying any texts; styles and contents vary, and each should be promotive of your learning. We have included a brief overview of each text reference.

1. Abramson JH: *Survey Methods in Community Medicine.* Edinburgh and London, Churchill Livingston, 1974. First-class text in paperback, with many good chapters on topics not covered by other texts, such as constructing questionnaires, coding, planning records, pretests, and report writing. Very enjoyable reading and most promotive of learning.

2. Abramson JH, Terespolsky L, Brook JG, Kark SL: Cornell medical index as a health measure in epidemiological studies. *Brit J Prev Soc Med* 19:103–110, 1965.

3. Armitage P: *Statistical Methods in Medical Research.* Oxford, Blackwell Scientific Publications, 1971. Excellent text on statistical methods used in health research. A standard reference, it requires a working knowledge of some mathematical/statistical foundations; it probably is best suited for the advanced student.

4. Austin D, Werner SB: *Epidemiology for the Health Sciences: A Primer on Epidemiologic Concepts and Their Uses.* Springfield, Ill, Charles C Thomas, 1974. Very introductory paperback of 75 pages; touches upon most epidemiologic methods; easy to read.

5. Barker DJP, Rose G: *Epidemiology in Medical Practice.* London, Churchill Livingston, 1976. Paperback covering a number of basic epidemiological concepts with examples from United Kingdom. Application of epidemiology to description, prevention, and patient care of diseases is well presented.

6. Barker DJP: *Practical Epidemiology.* Edinburgh and London, Churchill Livingstone, 1973. Small paperback briefly covering epidemiological and some related statistical concepts in an applied context; easy to read.

7. Berkson J: Limitations of the application of fourfold table analysis to hospital data. *Biometrics Bull* 2:47–53, 1946.

8. Billewicz WZ: Matched samples in medical investigations. *Brit J Prev Soc Med* 18:167–173, 1964.

9. Bross IDJ: How case-for-case matching can improve design efficiency. *Am J Epid* 89:359–363, 1969.

10. Bross IDJ: Right answers from wrong assumptions. *Prev Med* 5:203–206, 1976.

11. Brown GW: Berkson fallacy revisited. Arch Am J Dis *Children* 130:56–60, 1976.

12. Buck C: Popper's philosophy for epidemiologists. *Int J Epid* 4:159–168,

13. Clark DW, MacMahon B (eds): *Preventive Medicine.* Boston, Little Brown & Co, 1967. A collection of 44 contributions covering many aspects of public health in addition to epidemiology and biostatistics. Chapters 4–7 on methods relevant to epidemiology are brief but excellent.

14. Clark V, Hopkins C: Time is of the essence. *J Chron Dis* 20:565–569, 1967.

15. Cole P, MacMahon B: Attributable risk percent in case-control studies. *Brit J Prev Soc Med* 25:242–244, 1971.

16. Colton T: *Statistics in Medicine.* Boston, Little Brown & Co, 1974. Available as a paperback, it is an easy-to-read introduction to statistics in medicine and other health sciences. Contents are very well presented and it contains good considerations of fallacies and reading the literature, among other relevant topics.

17. Cox A, Rutter M, Yule B, Quinton D: Bias resulting from missing information: some epidemiological findings. *Brit J Prev Soc Med* 31:131–136, 1977.

18. Deubner D, Tyroler HA, Cassell JC, Hames CG, Becker C: Attributable risk, population attributable risk, and population attributable fraction of death associated with hypertension in a biracial population. *Circulation* 52:901–908, 1975.

19. Dorn HF: Philosophy of inferences from retrospective studies. *Am J Pub Health* 43:677–683, 1953.

20. Duncan RC, Knapp RC, Miller, MC III: *Introductory Biostatistics for the Health Sciences.* New York, John Wiley & Sons, 1977. Paperback that presents relevant basic biostatistics in easy format. Ways of presenting data are covered well. Some ease with elementary mathematics/statistics is needed for maximal learning.

21. Durkheim E: *Suicide: A Study in Sociology*. Spaulding JA and Simpson G (trans). Glencoe, Ill, The Free Press, 1951. English translation of the classic study of suicide by a renowned French sociologist.

22. Epstein LM: Validity of a questionnaire for diagnosis of peptic ulcer in an ethnically heterogeneous population. *J Chronic Dis* 22:49–55, 1969.

23. Faris R, Dunham HW: *Mental Disorders in Urban Areas*. Chicago and London, The University of Chicago Press, 1939. A classic ecological study of schizophrenia and other psychoses, with fine chapters on bias and selection in epidemiology. It is available as paperback.

24. Feinstein AR: *Clinical Biostatistics*. St. Louis, The CV Mosby Co, 1977.

25. Fisher FD: *An Introduction to Epidemiology: A Programmed Text*. New York, Appelton-Century-Crofts, 1975. For those who enjoy programmed texts, this one is worth perusing. It covers most concepts and methods of epidemiology and their applications.

26. Fox J, Hall C, Elveback L: *Epidemiology: Man and Disease*. London, The MacMillan Co, 1970. Follows the traditional agent/host/environment format with scattered statistical chapters. Concentrates on infectious diseases, with good chapters on strategies, study design, and related statistics.

27. Friedman GD: *Primer of Epidemiology*, ed 2. New York, McGraw-Hill Book Co, 1980. Excellent, easy-to-read paperback that manages to effectively compress much information into 288 pages. It is used frequently by students.

28. Hill AB: The environment and disease: association or causation? *Proc Roy Soc of Med* 58:295–300, 1965.

29. Hill AB: *Principles of Medical Statistics*, ed 9. New York, Oxford University Press, 1971. Covers most commonly used biostatistical concepts and techniques in easy-to-follow manner. Excellent text for those who prefer nonmathematical presentation of material. (In a lecture, the eminent British biostatistician Sir Austin Hill referred to this book as 'statistics without tears"; he was not wrong.) It includes a worthwhile set of problems and explanations of solutions.

30. Hill AB: *Statistical Methods in Clinical and Preventive Medicine*. Edinburgh and London, E & S Livingstone Ltd, 1962. A compilation of superbly written papers containing descriptions of some classic studies, including the first clinical trial of streptomycin in the treatment of pulmonary tuberculosis. The range of topics includes important issues of substance, methods, and research on humans. It is out of print, but should be available in libraries.

31. Holland WW, Karhauser L (eds) assisted by Wainwright AH: *Health Care and Epidemiology*. London, Henry Kimpton Publishers, 1978. A compilation of presentations by a group of epidemiologists from many countries. They include methods and other selected aspects such as the use of registers in the study of diseases.

32. Huff D: *How to Lie with Statistics.* New York, WW Norton & Co, 1954. An oldie, but goodie on how statistics are misused in everyday living. Paperback—142 pages of light, pleasurable reading.

33. Jackson M: Against Popperized epidemiology. *Int J Epid* 5:9–11, 1976.

34. Kerlinger F: *Foundations of Behavioral Research,* ed 2. New York, Holt Rinehart & Winston, 1973. Covers research designs, measurement theory, data collection, and statistical techniques. Good treatment, although somewhat advanced.

35. Kessler II, Levin M (eds): *The Community as an Epidemiologic Laboratory.* Baltimore, Johns Hopkins Press, 1970. A compilation of excellent studies, illustrating epidemiological applications in research and health services.

36. Lilienfeld AM, Lilienfeld DE: *Foundations of Epidemiology.* New York, Oxford University Press, 1980. Available in paperback, this is an excellent addition to the available texts. Written by a renowned American epidemiologist and his son, it deals with many aspects of epidemiology, including methods. Statistical examples require some ease with mathamatics/statistics.

37. Linder FE, Grove RD: Techniques of vital statistics. *Vital Statistics Rates in the US 1900–1940,* Department of Health, Education, and Welfare, US Public Health Service, National Center for Health Statistics, 1965, chap 1–4. An excellent publication from the National Center for Health Statistics that illustrates many statistical techniques.

38. MacMahon B, Pugh TF: *Epidemiology: Principles and Methods.* Boston, Little, Brown & Co, 1970. This excellent book is used by most professional epidemiology students and faculty. One of the best references on methods and concepts, it has withstood the tests of time and use.

39. Mainland D: The risk of fallacious conclusions from autopsy data on the incidence of diseases with applications to heart disease. *Am Heart J* 45:644–654, 1953.

40. Mausner JS, Bahn AK: *Epidemiology: An Introductory Text.* Philadelphia, WB Saunders Co, 1974. This text covers basics, including most aspects of methods used in epidemiology with relevant biostatistics. Excellent easy-to-use text for beginners; it specifically considers the relationship of epidemiology to infectious and to chronic disease. Includes self-evaluation questions.

41. Maxcy KF (ed): *Papers of Wade Hampton Frost.* New York and London, Oxford University Press, 1941. Textbook containing descriptions of Frost's classic studies. Available in libraries.

42. Medalie JH, Riss E, Neufeld HN, Kahn HA, Perlstein T, Balogh M, Baruch D, Sive P, Goldburdt UM: Some practical problems of observer variation in a large survey in Eliakim M, Newfield HM (eds): *Cardiology: Current Topics and Progress.* New York and London, Academic Press, 1970, pp 100–104.

43. Miettinen O: Confounding and effect-modification. *Am J Epid*, 100:350–353, 1974.

44. Miettinen O: Matching and design efficiency in retrospective studies. *Am J Epid* 91:111–118, 1970.

45. Morris JN: *Uses of Epidemiology*, ed 3. Edinburgh and London, E & S Livingston Ltd, 1975. Excellent, easy-to-read book, concentrating on uses and applications of epidemiology rather than on methods. This is one of the few books directly addressing the uses of epidemiology; it does include some methods and concepts. Available in paperback.

46. Morton RF, Hekel JR: *A Study Guide to Epidemiology and Biostatistics, Including 100 Multiple Choice Questions*. Baltimore, University Park Press, 1979. A short guide that touches upon a number of concepts and methods, and presents self-evaluation questions on each. Good guide for rapid study and revision.

47. Peterson DR, Thomas DB: *Fundamentals of Epidemiology, An Instruction Manual*. Lexington, Mass, Lexington Books, 1979. A 93-page paperback text that presents a quick overview of a number of concepts. Includes a series of text problems and answers.

48. Platt J: Strong inference. *Science* 146:347–353, 1964.

49. Roberts RS, Spitzer WO, Delmore T, Sackett DL: An empirical demonstration of Berkson's bias. *J Chron Dis*, 31:119–128, 1978.

50. Rothman KJ: A pictorial representation of confounding in epidemiologic studies. *J Chron Dis* 28:101–108, 1975.

51. Rothman J: Causes. *Am J Epid* 104:587–592, 1976.

52. Rothman KJ: Epidemiologic methods in clinical trials. *Cancer* 39:1771–1775, 1977.

53. Runyon R, Haber A: *Fundamentals of Behavioral Statistics*, ed 3. Reading, Mass, Addison-Wesley Publishing Co, 1976. Fine text with good student workbook. Fairly easy to use, though requires some ease with mathematics. Illustrates frequently used statistical techniques.

54. Schilling R, Hughes JPW, Dingwall-Fordyce I: Disagreement between observers in an epidemiological study of respiratory disease. *Brit Med J* 1:65–68, 1955.

55. Slonim MJ: *Sampling*. New York, Simon & Schuster, 1960. An elementary, nonmathematical discussion of the different sampling techniques, including simple random sampling, stratified sampling, cluster sampling, and systematic sampling. It is oriented primarily toward business applications of sampling, but is general enough to appeal to almost anyone. Paperback, 145 pages.

56. Smith A: Epidemiological reasoning, comments on Popper's philosophy for epidemiologists by Carol Buck, *Int J Epid* 4:169–172, 1975.

57. Snow J: *On the Mode of Communication of Cholera*, ed 2. London, J & A Churchill Ltd, 1855. Reproduced in Richardson BW: *Snow on Cholera*. New York, The Commonwealth Fund, 1936.

58. The Steering Committee: The hypertension detection and follow-up program, in Paul O (ed): *Epidemiology and Control of Hypertension*, New York, Stratton International Medical Book Corp, 1974, pp 663–670.

59. Susser M: Judgment and causal inference: criteria in epidemiologic studies. *Am J Epid* 105:1–15, 1977.

60. Swinson TDV: *Statistics at Square One*. London, British Medical Assoc, 1976. Compilation of a series of articles published in the *BritishMedical Journal*. In this 86-page paperback, the main statistical concepts are presented very well indeed.

61. Taylor I, Knowelden J: *Principles of Epidemiology*, ed 2. London, J & A Churchill Ltd, 1964. Although not widely used in the United States, this book contains good coverage of many epidemiological principles in understandable, not heavily mathematical formats. Lacks updating of newer methods.

62. Taylor JW: Simple estimation of population attributable risk from case-control studies. *Am J Epid* 106:260, 1977.

63. Tyroler HA, Heyden S, Hames CG: Weight and hypertension: Evans County studies of Blacks and Whites, in Paul O (ed): *Epidemiology and Control of Hypertension*, New York, Stratton International Medical Book Corp, 1975, pp. 177–204.

64. *Vital Statistics of the United States, 1970*, vol 2, Mortality, parts A and B. US Dept of Health, Education, and Welfare, Public Health Service, National Center for Health Statistics, 1974. This is an illustration of the excellent sets of series of data available from the National Center for Health Statistics. (We strongly recommend that you request being put on the center's mailing list.)

65. Walter S: Calculation of attributable risks from epidemiological data. *Int J Epid* 7:175–182, 1978.

66. Warwick DP, Lininger CA: *The Sample Survey: Theory and Practice*. New York, McGraw-Hill Book Co, 1975. Paperback with excellent coverage of steps in doing a survey, designing a questionnaire, conducting an interview, editing and coding responses on questionnaires, and doing analysis.

67. White KL, Henderson MM (eds): *Epidemiology as a Fundamental Science: Its Uses in Health Services Planning, Administration, and Evaluation*. New York, Oxford University Press, 1976. A report of an international conference that addressed the application of epidemiology to health sciences, including health manpower training. It does not cover epidemiologic or related statistical methods or principles.

68. Witts LJ (ed): *Medical Surveys and Clinical Trials*, ed 2. New York and Toronto, Oxford University Press, 1964. This text by greats in British medical care epidemiological circles is not widely advertised or used in the United States, but it is excellent. Chapters 1–9 are well written and relevant to epidemiological methods. It is of particular interest to clinically oriented professionals interested in epidemiology.

Self-Evaluation Problems

These problems are included in this manual to permit you to evaluate your learning. Explanations of our thinking about them and our suggested correct interpretations are included in Appendix B. We suggest you record your own responses before checking the answers. You should regard all the examples as hypothetical.

Additional self-evaluation problems can be found in the books listed in the references at the end of these problems.

1. Suppose a new drug is discovered that is highly effective in the treatment of a form of cancer that previously had been rapidly fatal. Which of the following rates will be *least* affected by the widespread use of the drug? (Check one.)

a._____ Five-year survival rate for this type of cancer
b._____ Prevalence rate for this type of cancer
c._____ Incidence rate for this type of cancer
d._____ Mortality rate for this type of cancer

2. In a study concerned with the possible effects of air pollution on the development of chronic bronchitis, the following data were obtained.

> A population of 9,000 White men aged 45 years was examined in January 1960. Of these, 6,000 lived in areas that exposed them to air pollution and 3,000 did not. At this examination, 90 cases of chronic bronchitis were discovered, 60 among those exposed to air pollution.
>
> All the men initially examined who did not have chronic bronchitis were available for subsequent repeated examinations over the next five years.

These revealed 268 new cases of chronic bronchitis in the total group, including 30 among those not exposed to air pollution.

The prevalence rates of chronic bronchitis in January 1960 were:

	Numerator	Denominator		Prevalence rate/1,000
a.	_____	_____	Among those exposed to air pollution	_____
b.	_____	_____	Among those not exposed to air pollution	_____

The incidence rates of chronic bronchitis over the five years were:

	Numerator	Denominator		Incidence rate/1,000
c.	_____	_____	Among those exposed to air pollution	_____
d.	_____	_____	Among those not exposed to air pollution	_____
e.	_____	_____	In the total sample	_____

f. Which of the following conclusions can be drawn from the *prevalence* data? (Check one.)

_____(1) Air pollution is associated with chronic bronchitis.
_____(2) Air pollution is not associated with chronic bronchitis.

g. Which of the following conclusions can be drawn from the *incidence* data? (Check one.)

_____(1) Air pollution is associated with chronic bronchitis.
_____(2) Air pollution is not associated with chronic bronchitis.

In order to determine whether air pollution is or is not causally related to chronic bronchitis, the possibility that the conclusions, drawn from either the prevalence or the incidence data, may be artifactual (spurious) has to be considered. Three of the more common sources of spurious conclusions are: selective survival, selective migration, and secondary association (due to confounding variables).
For each source of spurious conclusion, indicate whether it is more likely to apply to the prevalence data, to the incidence data, or equally to both sets of data. (Check the *one best* answer for each.)

h. Selective survival is:
_____(1) More likely to have influenced the conclusions drawn from the prevalence data than from the incidence data

_____(2) More likely to have influenced the conclusions drawn from the incidence data than from the prevalence data

_____(3) Equally likely to have influenced the conclusions drawn from the prevalence or the incidence data

i. Selective migration is:

_____(1) More likely to have influenced the conclusions drawn from the prevalence data than from the incidence data

_____(2) More likely to have influenced the conclusions drawn from the incidence data than from the prevalence data

_____(3) Equally likely to have influenced the conclusions drawn from the prevalence or the incidence data

j. Secondary (artifactual) associations are:

_____(1) More likely to have influenced the conclusions drawn from the prevalence data than from the incidence data

_____(2) More likely to have influenced the conclusions drawn from the incidence data than from the prevalence data

_____(3) Equally likely to have influenced the conclusions drawn from the prevalence or the incidence data

3. Death rates from all causes are reported to be lower in professional and managerial occupations than in unskilled occupations. You would suspect this association between occupational status and death to be secondary (due to confounding variables) if you knew the following facts. (Check as many as would make you suspect a secondary association.)

a._____ People in unskilled occupations are older than those in professional and managerial occupations.

b._____ People in professional and managerial occupations are older than those in unskilled occupations.

c._____ Professional and managerial occupations contain a greater proportion of women than do unskilled occupations.

d._____ There are more people in unskilled occupations than there are in professional and managerial occupations.

4. A health agency was concerned with two problems: the high rate of recurrence of rheumatic heart disease in children with rheumatic fever and the high rate of complications occurring in children with diabetes. The consequences (in terms of subsequent disability and death) of rheumatic fever recurrences and diabetic complications are equally serious. Furthermore, the prevalences of diabetes and rheumatic heart disease were the same in the population for which the agency was responsible.

       The high rate of recurrence of rheumatic heart disease was due to the failure of many children with rheumatic fever to take their penicillin regularly. The high rate of diabetic complications was due to failure of diabetic children to take insulin regularly. To reduce these problems the agency wished to try two approaches; the first was sending a postcard each month to the families to remind them the patient must have penicillin or insulin regularly. The second was a regular home visit by a nurse. For this purpose, they drew a random sample of their rheumatic fever patients and a similar sample of their juvenile diabetic patients. One third of each sample received no intervention, one third of each sample received a regular postcard, and one third a home visit.

As can be seen from Tables A.1 and A.2, which were compiled one year after the trials started, sending a postcard had little effect, but home visits were highly effective for both rheumatic fever and diabetes.

Table A.1   **Recurrence of Rheumatic Heart Disease in Children with Rheumatic Fever**

Method of intervention	Recurrences of rheumatic heart disease/1,000
No intervention	15.7
Regular postcard	15.5
Home visits	5.0

Table A.2   **Occurrences of Diabetic Complications in Diabetic Children**

Method of intervention	Diabetic complications/1,000
No intervention	4.5
Regular postcard	4.2
Home visits	0.5

As a result of this information it was decided to make home visiting a routine program of the agency. Due to personal shortage, however, such home visits could only be made to all rheumatic fever patients or to all diabetic patients (but *not* to both). On the basis of the data presented in Tables A.1 and A.2, which condition should receive the home visits? (Check one.)

a._____ Rheumatic fever children

b._____ Diabetic children

Show the data from which you drew your conclusions.

5. A study was undertaken to evaluate the effectiveness of a prenatal program. An objective of this program was to reduce the perinatal mortality rate (rate of deaths of infants in first seven days of life).

Two populations were studied: (1) all primigravidae (with first pregnancy) aged 20 to 24 who attended the clinic for prenatal care during a particular year and (2) a representative sample of primigravidae from the community served by the clinic who were pregnant during this same period and who received no prenatal care. This sample was of the same age and ethnic group as the attenders.

The results were as shown in Tables A.3 and A.4.

Table A.3   ***Perinatal Mortality Rates in Women Receiving and Not Receiving Prenatal Care***

Prenatal care at clinic	No. of Women	Perinatal deaths	Perinatal mortality rate/1,000
Receiving pre- natal care	200	5	25.0
No prenatal care	150	10	66.7
Total	350	15	42.9

Table A.4   ***Perinatal Mortality Rates***
by Educational Level of Women

Education	No. of Women	Perinatal deaths	Perinatal mortality rate/1,000
High school graduates	190	6	31.6
Non-high school graduates	160	9	56.3
Total	350	15	42.9

If you knew that 110 of the women who had received prenatal care were high school graduates and that two of them had had an infant that died in the perinatal period (and assuming that all the results are statistically significant), what would you conclude from these data? (Check as many as are correct.)

a._____ That primigravidae aged 20 to 24 who received perinatal care had a reduced perinatal mortality rate compared to those receiving no prenatal care.

b._____ That the prenatal program had *not* been effective. The reduction in perinatal mortality rate was not due to the program but due to the higher educational level of the woman using the program.

c._____ That prenatal care was beneficial for more educated mothers but did not help less educated mothers in this country.

d._____ That in this county, the higher rates of perinatal mortality in less educated as compared with more educated women were due also to some factors over and above the lack of prenatal care.

Present the complete table from which you drew you conclusions.

6. To determine whether a newly invented birth control pill increased the risk of stroke, a cohort study was started. A random sample of women of child-bearing age was selected and examined to make sure that none had any evidence of stroke; 9,920 individuals were thus identified as being eligible for study. Of these, 1,000 were taking the birth control pill regularly and the remainder were not taking it at all. The entire sample was followed for ten years with the results shown in Table A.5.

Table A.5   **New Cases of Stroke Over Ten Years by Pill-Taking Status**

	New cases of stroke over ten years	Free of stroke over ten years	Total
Women taking pill	10	990	1,000
Women not taking pill	10	8,910	8,920
Total	20	9,900	9,920

From these data, which of the following conclusions can be drawn? (Check the one best answer.)

a._____ Taking the pill *does* increase the risk of stroke and the degree of this risk is shown by the fact that 10/1,000 (1%) of those taking the pill developed a stroke, whereas only 10/8,920 (0.1%) of those not taking the pill developed a stroke.

b._____ Taking the pill *does not* increase the risk of stroke because 50% (10/20) of stroke cases were taking the pill and 50% (10/20) of stroke cases were not taking the pill.

c._____ Taking the pill *does not* increase the risk of stroke because although 10/1,000 (1%) of those taking the pill did develop a stroke, 990/1,000 (99%) of those also taking the pill did not develop a stroke.

d._____ Taking the pill *does* increase the risk of stroke and the degree of this risk is shown by the fact that 10/20 (50%) of the stroke cases were taking the pill, whereas only 990/9,900 (10%) of those free of stroke were taking the pill.

7. In order to determine whether exposure to various industrial pollutants increased the risk of lung cancer, the average annual death rates for lung cancer over a ten-year period were analyzed for male employees in five different sorts of industries. These industries are labeled A–E in Table A.6. (Because lung cancer is almost invariably fatal and there is a short interval between diagnosis and death, death rates are good approximations of incidence.)

Table A.6   **Average Annual Death Rate for Lung Cancer for Male Employees by Industry, 1960–1969**

Industry	Death rate per 100,000 employees
A	72
B	71
C	50
D	49
E	49

The death rates in industries A and B were higher than those in C, D, and E. (The differences were statistically significant.) It was known, however, that both the age distribution and cigarette-smoking patterns differed in those different industries. Because both age and cigarette smoking increase the risk of lung cancer, it was necessary to control for these before concluding that some factor in industries A and B was responsible for an increased risk of lung cancer. To control for them, an age and cigarette smoking standardized mortality ratio (SMR) was computed. The results were as shown in Table A.7.

Table A.7   **Standardized Mortality Ratio for Lung Cancer for Male Employees by Industry, 1960–1969**

Industry	SMR
A	180.6
B	101.1
C	210.2
D	98.9
E	101.3

From these data, which of the following conclusions can be drawn? (Check as many as may be true.)

a._____ Some factors in industries A and C were probably increasing the risk of lung cancer.

b._____ These data show that neither cigarette smoking nor age was related to lung cancer in industries B, D, and E.

c._____ Industry B must have had either more cigarette smokers and/ or older employees than industry C.

8. For a particular county, all mothers giving birth to a first child during a particular year were classified by place of residence (urban or rural) and by social class. The *mean birthweights* of the babies were tabulated as shown in Table A.8.

Table A.8   **Mean Birthweights in Grams by Maternal Place of Residence and Social Class**

	Place of residence		
Social class	Rural	Urban	All places
Low	3,300	3,309	3,303
High	3,672	3,669	3,671
All Classes	3,364	3,592	3,475

If these data were available and a new investigation were being planned to search for the causes of low birthweight, how would it be most logical to start this search? (Check the one best answer.)

a._____ By attempting to identify the relevant factors in rural way of living as contrasted to urban.

b._____ By attempting to identify the relevant factors in the way of life of lower-class people as compared with higher-class people.

c._____ By attempting to identify the relevant factors that distinguish rural from urban people *and* low from high social class.

d._____ To ignore both place of residence and social class status as neither of these are associated with birthweight.

9. Sensitivity and specificity are useful indices in the evaluation of a newly developed screening test. Table A.9 represents the evaluation of a screening test for a particular disease against a well-established method of diagnosing that disease. A, B, C, and D represent frequencies.

Table A.9   *Presence and Absence of Disease by Screening Test and by Established Method*

	According to the well-established method	
According to the screening test	Disease present	Disease absent
Disease present	A	B
Disease absent	C	D

a. The *sensitivity* of the screening test may be defined as (check one):

_____(1) C / (C + D)
_____(2) C / (A + C)
_____(3) A / (A + C)
_____(4) A / (A + B)

b. The specificity of the screening test may be defined as (check one):

_____(1) D / (C + D)
_____(2) D / (A + D)
_____(3) D / (B + D)
_____(4) None of the above.

c. The frequency that represents the *false positives* of the screening test is (check one):

_____(1) A
_____(2) B
_____(3) C
_____(4) D

10. For a disease that is known to be spread by food and water, the data in Table A.10 were available for a particular county.

Table A.10 **Number of New Cases, All Cases and Deaths of Disease by Year**

Year	Population of county	New cases	All cases	Deaths
1955	50,000	100	200	5
1960	75,000	150	225	5
1965	100,000	200	250	5

Assuming that the data in the table were accurate and complete, which of the following would you regard them as suggestive evidence of? (Check one.)

a._____ A successful environmental health program; that is, improvement in the sanitary quality of food and water.

b._____ Improvement in treatment of the disease.

c._____ A successful environmental health program *and* improvement in treatment.

d._____ None of the above.

11. For each question, check the one numbered heading that is most closely related to it.

a. Evaluation of a newly developed procedure against a standard procedure.

_____(1) Validity
_____(2) Reliability
_____(3) Both
_____(4) Neither

b. Comparisons of responses to a newly developed questionnaire obtained one month apart.

_____(1) Validity
_____(2) Reliability
_____(3) Both
_____(4) Neither

c. Expressed as sensitivity and specificity.

_____(1) Validity
_____(2) Reliability
_____(3) Both
_____(4) Neither

12. For each of the circumstances listed below check which study method applies.

a. A study concerned with a rare disease.

_____(1) Case-control
_____(2) Cohort

b. A study that attempted to determine whether a high absenteeism rate in school children led to poor grades or whether poor grades led to high absenteeism.

_____(1) Case-control
_____(2) Cohort

c. A study in which selective survival could seriously bias the results.

_____(1) Case-control
_____(2) Cohort

d. A study in which it was important to quantify the attributable risk of the characteristic.

_____(1) Case-control
_____(2) Cohort

e. A study in which the latent or determination period between exposure to the characteristic and the onset of the condition (or determination) might be as long as 20 years.

_____(1) Case-control
_____(2) Cohort

13.

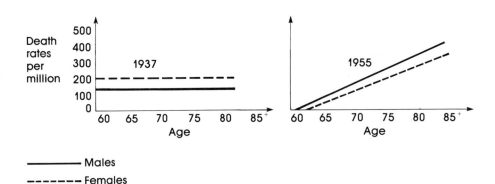

Figure A.1 Death rates from appendicitis by age and sex in the United States, 1937 and 1955.

Which of the following explanations could account for the phenomenon in Figure A.1? (Check as many as are correct.)

a._____ Improvements in treatment between 1937 and 1955 may have benefited the younger of the age groups more than the older.

b._____ Bias in diagnosing causes of death at different ages.

c._____ Selective migration to Europe in 1945 of younger couples with low risk of death from appendicitis.

d._____Changes in the numbers of people of these different ages in the population at the two points in time.

14. Two cohort studies on coronary heart disease have recently published their results. One was conducted in Framingham, Massachusetts and the other in Puerto Rico. The methods used in each study were identical and standardized criteria for diagnoses were used. Some of the results are shown in Table A.11.

Table A.11 **Prevalence and Incidence of Coronary Heart Disease in Men aged 60–64, Framingham and Puerto Rico, 1960–1970**

	Prevalence/ 100,000 (1970)	Average incidence/ 100,000 (1960–1970)
Framingham	37.4	27.0
Puerto Rico	15.5	5.2

There was minimal (and approximately equal) attrition in both studies over the course of time the studies were conducted, and no known cure for coronary heart disease exists.

From these data would you infer that the death rate from coronary heart disease in men of this age was (check one):

a._____ Higher in Framingham than in Puerto Rico

b._____ Higher in Puerto Rico than Framingham

c._____ Equal in Framingham and Puerto Rico

15. In the continuing controversy over the role of cigarette smoking as a cause of lung cancer, an investigator makes the following statement.

> There are certain well-known data that refute the hypothesis that cigarette smoking is a cause of lung cancer. For example in Great Britain the *per capita* consumption of cigarettes is half as much as in the United States, but the incidence of lung cancer is twice as much. In Australia the *per capita* consumption of cigarettes is about the same as in Great Britain, yet Australians have half as much lung cancer. In Holland the *per capita* consumption of cigarettes is lower than the United States but there is 33% more lung cancer.

> What reasoning would lead you to agree or disagree with the investigator that these data refute the hypothesis that cigarette smoking causes lung cancer? (Check the one best answer.)

a._____ Disagree with the investigator because the populations of the countries mentioned vary so much in size.

b._____ Agree with the investigator but *only* if there is good evidence that there was no bias in the diagnosis of lung cancer (if the criteria for diagnosing lung cancer were the same in each country).

c._____ Disagree with the investigator because this is an example of the ecologic fallacy.

d._____ Disagree with the investigator because he is basing his comparisons on numerator data only.

16. In a study of broken appointments among patients attending a clinic, the effect of distance from the clinic was examined. Part of the results was as shown in Table A.12.

Table A.12   Rate of Broken Appointments by Distance Patients Live from Clinic, for Women, Aged 45–49

Miles from clinic	% broken appointments
10 or greater	53
5–9	47
1–4	39
less than one	29

These differences were statistically significant. It was suspected, however, that the social class composition of the patients living at different distances from the clinic differed, and thus might have affected their broken appointments. Accordingly, to control for social class, each patient was given a social class score, and a *social class adjusted* rate of broken appointments was computed, as shown in Table A.13.

Table A.13   **Rate of Broken Appointments Adjusted for Social Class by Distance Patients Live from Clinic, for Women, Aged 45–49**

Miles from clinic	% broken appointments
10 or greater	42
5–9	44
1–4	40
less than one	41

These adjusted rates were not statistically significantly different from each other.

From these data, which of the following conclusions can be drawn (in each case the conclusions would be restricted to females aged 45 to 49)? (Check as many as are correct.)

a._____ The social class adjusted results decrease the likelihood that distance from the clinic was related causally to broken appointments.

b._____ The social class adjusted results decrease the likelihood that social class was related to broken appointments.

c._____ The data confirm that the *social class distribution* of patients living at different distances from the clinic does differ.

d._____ The data increase the likelihood that *both distance from the clinic* and *social class* of the patients were related to broken appointments.

17. As an administrator of a chronic disease control program, you have two screening tests available to you for the early detection of a particular disease. Screening test A has a sensitivity of 95% and a specificity of 70%. Screening test B has a sensitivity of 60% and a specificity of 90%. Given the following circumstances, which test would you choose? (Check A or B for each circumstance.)

a. If the disease were one whose presence caused a high level of anxiety, and to avoid needless emotional suffering you wanted to reduce the probability of suggesting to healthy people that they had the disease. _____ A _____ B

b. If the most important concern were not to overburden the health care system with unnecessary referrals for further diagnostic workups following the screening. _____ A _____ B

c. If this were a treatable disease in its early stages but more fatal if not detected early. _____ A _____ B

d. If this were a highly infectious disease in its early stages, but less infectious in later stages and you needed to protect the public from contact with the infectious stage of the disease. _____ A _____ B

18. Two observers each examined independently the same 100 subjects. Each observer reported the prevalence of diabetes as 25% in the sample. Present a table demonstrating how it is possible for observer 1 and observer 2 to have interobserver reliability of only 50% despite their identical estimates of prevalence.

19. As part of a cancer control program, a state's Department of Human Services started a program in 1960 to reduce the exposure of the population to X rays. To help evaluate the effectiveness of the program, a statewide cancer register was developed so that all newly diagnosed cases of cancer could be recorded. The data in Table A.14 refer to a specific form of cancer in children (aged 0 to 4) in which exposure to X rays is thought to be particularly important as part of the cause, and for which there is no cure.

Table A.14   **Total Number of Children Aged 0–4,**
Number of New Cases and Number of Cases on
Register, by Year

Year	Children aged 0–4 in the state	Newly diagnosed cases of Cancer	Cancer cases on register
1960	100,000	100	200
1965	150,000	120	350
1970	200,000	130	550

Assume that the reporting of new cases was reasonably complete and that there had been minimal in- or out-migration from the state during this ten-year period. Assume, also, that in the neighboring states that had not had such a program none of the cancer rates (for this particular form of cancer in this age group) had changed in this ten-year period. What would you regard these data as suggesting (insofar as this particular cancer in this age group was concerned)? (Check the one best answer.)

a._____ The program to prevent cancer had *not* been successful, but there had been an improvement in the ability to treat cancer during this period.

b._____ The program to prevent cancer had been successful but there had been no improvement in the ability to treat cancer.

c._____ The program had been successful in preventing cancer *and* there had been an improvement in the ability to treat cancer.

d._____ Neither had the program to prevent cancer been successful *nor* had there been any improvement in treatment.

20. In a recent article on lead poisoning in children, the authors wrote about their study of 136 children with lead poisoning reported by all hospitals in Cleveland between 1963 and 1969. The data in Tables A.15 and A.16 were presented.

On the basis of these data, the authors concluded that:

1. The most vulnerable age for lead poisoning is between 1 and 3.5 years (12–42 months).

2. Hospital admissions for lead poisoning occur more during the summer months than at any other time.

Table A.15   *Distribution of Lead Poisoning*
in Children by Age, 1963–1969

Age in months	Cases of lead poisoning
9 and under	0
10–12	3
13–18	25
19–24	39
25–30	30
31–36	17
37–42	13
43–48	4
49 and over	4
Unknown	1
Total	136

Table A.16   *Months of First Admission of 136*
Lead-Poisoned Children in Cleveland, 1963–1969

Month	Cases admitted
January	3
February	5
March	2
April	5
May	12
June	19
July	32
August	28
September	15
October	9
November	4
December	2
Total	136

For each conclusion, check the one best answer.

Conclusion 1 (The most vulnerable age is between 1 and 3.5 years.)

a._____ Disagree with the conclusion because this is an example of the ecologic fallacy.

b._____ Disagree with the conclusion because it is based upon numerator data only.

c._____ Agree with the conclusion but only if there has been no bias in the diagnosis of lead poisoning.

d._____ Disagree with the conclusion because the antecedent-consequent relationship cannot be determined from this study design.

Conclusion 2 (Hospital admissions occur more during the summer months.)

a._____ Disagree with the conclusion because this is an example of the ecologic fallacy.

b._____ Disagree with the conclusion because it is based upon numerator data only.

c._____ Agree with the conclusion but only if there has been no bias in the diagnosis of lead poisoning.

d._____ Disagree with the conclusion because the antecedent-consequent relationship cannot be determined from this study design.

21. The data in Table A.17 were reported from a cohort study conducted on some professional male workers.

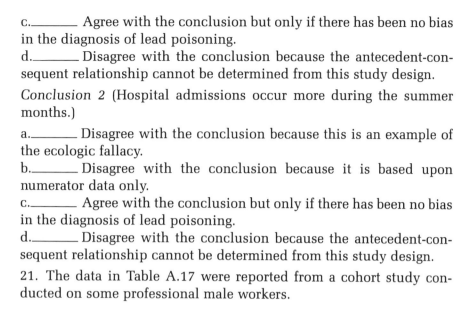

Table A.17   Age-Adjusted Mortality Rates from Lung Cancer and Coronary Heart Disease for Heavy Cigarette Smokers and Nonsmokers

Annual age-adjusted death rate/100,000 men

	Lung cancer	CHD
Heavy smokers	160	599
Nonsmokers	7	422

The results indicate (check *as many* as are correct and show the figures upon which you based your conclusions):

a._____ More workers would be saved from lung cancer than coronary disease if no one smoked.

b._____ More workers would be saved from coronary heart disease than from lung cancer if no one smoked.

c._____ Heavy smoking carries a higher relative risk for lung cancer than for CHD.

d._____ Heavy smoking carries a higher relative risk for CHD than for lung cancer.

22. In a cohort study concerned with the incidence of stroke in rural and urban men, the data in Tables A.18 and A.19 were presented. The study was well conducted. Diagnostic criteria were well standardized (no bias), the samples were representative, and there was minimal attrition (no selection). Differences were statistically significant.

From these data, what would the most appropriate conclusion be? (Check the one best answer.)

a._____ In this sample, the higher incidence rates in rural men indicate some increased risk (other than age) associated with rural living.

b._____ In this sample, there is an increased risk (other than age) associated with urban living because at each age the urban incidence rates are higher than the rural.

c._____ No comparison of urban versus rural rates can be made from these tables because there are nearly twice as many urban as rural men at risk.

d._____ Some error in assigning ages must have been made in this study because although the total rates (Table A.18) are higher in rural men, when the two populations are broken down into age groups (Table A.19), the urban rates are always higher than the rural at each age group.

Table A.18   **Incidence of Stroke in Rural and Urban Men**

	Rural men	Urban men
Population at risk	529	937
Cases of stroke	24	41
Incidence rate per 1,000	45.3	43.8

Table A.19   **Incidence of Stroke in Rural and Urban Men, by Age**

	Rural			Urban		
Age	PAR	Cases of stroke	Incidence rate/1,000	PAR	Cases of stroke	Incidence rate/1,000
35–44	147	1	6.8	436	6	13.8
45–54	87	3	34.5	188	7	37.2
55–64	133	4	30.1	195	13	66.7
65–74	160	16	100.0	103	15	145.6
Unknown	2	0	—	15	0	—
Total	529	24		937	41	

23. In an attempt to determine the effect of driver education on automobile accidents, a case-control study was undertaken. One-hundred-fifty individuals between the ages of 16 and 25 who had been responsible for an automobile accident were suitably matched with 300 controls who had had no accident. The "exposure," or number of miles driven, was the same in the two groups. The analyses were performed separately for females and males. Differences were statistically significant. On the basis of the data in Table A.20, the investigators drew the

Table A.20   ***Driver Education and Automobile Accidents in Cases and Controls***

Driver education	Females		Males	
	Accident cases	No accident	Accident cases	No accident
Had driver education	10	50	60	120
Did not have driver education	40	50	40	280
Total	50	100	100	200

following conclusions. *For females:* "There is an association between lack of driver education and accidents because the majority of the accident cases did not have driver education." *For males:* "In males, however, the opposite association exists because the majority of the accident cases *did* have driver education."

a. As far as females are concerned, would you (check the one best answer):

———(1) Disagree with the investigators' conclusions even *though* they *did* make the correct comparisons.

———(2) Agree with the investigators' conclusions even *though* they *did not* make the appropriate comparisons.

———(3) Disagree with the investigators' conclusions *because* they *did not* make the appropriate comparisons.

———(4)Agree with the investigators' conclusions *because* they *did* make the appropriate comparisons.

b. Give the numerators and denominators of the rates or proportions you used to arrive at your answer.

c. As far as males are concerned, would you (check the one best answer):

———(1) Disagree with the investigator's conclusions even *though* they *did* make the correct comparisons.

———(2) Agree with the investigator's conclusions even *though* they *did not* make the appropriate comparisons.

———(3) Disagree with the investigator's conclusions *because* they *did not* make the appropriate comparisons.

———(4) Agree with the investigator's conclusions *because* they *did* make the appropriate comparisons.

d. Give the numerators and denominators of the rates or proportions you used to arrive at your answer.

24. In a study to determine the relationship between physical activity and coronary heart disease, men of similar age and of the same ethnic

group in three different occupations were compared. The occupations were classified as physically active, intermediate activity, and sendentary. The findings were as shown in Table A.21.

Table A.21   ***Coronary Heart Disease, by Occupational Type***

Occupational type	No. of Men	Cases of CHD	Rate per 1,000
Active	6,000	20	3.3
Intermediate	3,000	30	10.0
Sedentary	1,000	20	20.0
Total	10,000	70	7.0

Questions (a) and (b) are true-false questions all relating to these data.

a. If the data shown in Table A.21 were from a *cross-sectional study* (prevalence data) and the differences were statistically significant, indicate whether *each* of the following statements would be *true* or *false*.

True _____
False _____
    (1) The associations shown in Table A.21 could have occurred if physical activity was protective against coronary heart disease.

True _____
False _____
    (2) The associations could be entirely a result of men with CHD changing occupations from active to more sendentary jobs.

True _____
False _____
    (3) The associations could be entirely a result of a higher case fatality in men in the active as compared with the sedentary jobs.

b. If the data shown in Table A.21 were from a *cohort study* (incidence data) and the differences were statistically significant, indicate whether *each* of the following statements would be *true* or *false*.

True _____
False _____
    (1) The associations shown in Table A.21 could have occurred if physical activity was protective against coronary heart disease.

True _____
False _____
    (2) The associations could be entirely a result of men with CHD changing occupations from active to more sedentary jobs.

True _____
False _____
    (3) The associations could be entirely a result of a higher case fatality in men in the active as compared with the sedentary jobs.

Answers and Explanations to Self-Evaluation Problems

B

1. The rate *least* affected would be the incidence rate, so (c) is correct answer. This is because treatment cannot affect the development of new cases (which is the incidence).

2. Prevalence rates in January 1960:

a. Among those exposed to air pollution = 60/6,000 = 10 per 1,000.
b. Among those *not* exposed to air pollution = 30/3,000 = 10 per 1,000.

Incidence rates over the five years:

c. Among those exposed to air pollution = 238/5,940 = 40.1 per 1,000 (note that the 60 cases prevalent in this group in 1960 are *not* at risk in incidence rates and so are excluded from the denominator).
d. Among those *not* exposed to air pollution = 30/2,970 = 10.1 per 1,000 (denominator reduced because 30 cases prevalent in 1960 not at risk in incidence).
e. In total sample = 268/8,910 (this is simple addition; do not just add the rates and divide by 2).
f. Correct answer is (2)—there is no difference in prevalence rates of exposed and not exposed groups.
g. Correct answer is (1)—incidence rate among the exposed is four times the rate among the nonexposed.
h. Correct answer is (1). Selective survival should not influence conclusions from the cohort study (which provides incidence data) because all subjects of the cohort are followed (even to death). Thus (2) and (3) are incorrect.
i. Correct answer is (1) for the same reasons as in (h).
j. Secondary associations due to confounding variables can be found in all study methods so (3) is correct answer.

3. a. Is correct because you know that age is associated with death, and the fact that people in unskilled occupations are older makes age a possible confounder.

b. Is incorrect because this says people in professional and managerial occupations are *older*; they are the group with the lower rates, so age is unlikely as a confounder.

c. This is correct if women have lower death rates (which they do); here sex is the suspected confounder.

d. Irrelevant because rates are compared.

4. Correct answer is (a). This is provided by calculating the relative risk of occurrence with no home visits, and the attributable risk with no home visits, for each disease as shown in Table B.1.

Table B.1   ***Relative Risk and Attributable Risk of Complications in Children with Rheumatic Fever or Diabetes***

	Relative risk with no home visits	Attributable risk with no home visits
Rheumatic fever recurrence	15.7/5.0 = 3.1	15.7 − 5.0 = 10.7 per 1,000
Diabetic complications	4.5/0.5 = 9.0	4.5 − 0.5 = 4 per 1,000

With home visits, rheumatic heart disease is relatively less likely (3.1 compared with 9) to reoccur than diabetes complications. However, home visits have a greater effect on preventing complications of rheumatic fever than diabetes (10.7 per 1,000 as compared with 4 per 1,000).

5. a. Correct. The perinatal mortality rate is lower in those who received prenatal care.

b. Incorrect. The difference in rates among those who received and those who did not receive care is found in both the less and the more educated women (the table controls for education levels).

c. Incorrect. The difference in rates among those who did and those who did not receive care is found among less educated women also.

d. Correct. Among those receiving care, the rate is higher among the less educated women.

Your table should resemble Table B.2. (For clarity the numerators and denominators were included; they all can be derived from the data given.)

Note: Even though the perinatal mortality rate is lower among those women who receive prenatal care, it is not certain that the prenatal care *caused* the reduced mortality. For example, if women chose

Table B.2   ***Perinatal Death Rates per 1,000 by Education and Prenatal Care, Primigravidae 20–24 Years Old***

	High school graduate	Non-high school graduate	Total
Prenatal care	(2/110) = 18.2	(3/90) = 33.3	(5/200) = 25.0
No prenatal care	(4/80) = 50.0	(6/70) = 85.7	(10/150) = 66.7
Total	(6/190) = 31.6	(9/160) = 56.3	(15/350) = 42.9

themselves to attend prenatal care, then the healthier women may have chosen prenatal care. If women had been randomly assigned in an experimental study to either prenatal or no prenatal care, then the cause-effect relationship could be argued with more persuasion.

6. Clearly we need to compare the incidence rates of stroke in pill takers and non-pill takers. These are 10/1,000 in pill takers and 10/8,920 in non-pill takers.

a. Is the only correct answer.
b. This comparison is incorrect and deals only with stroke victims (numerator data only).
c. The rate of non-pill takers developing stroke must be compared, not 990/1,000, which is the pill takers' rate of *not* developing stroke.
d. The decision is right about risk, but the comparisons made to support the decision are incorrect in a cohort study.

7. Correct answers are (a) and (c).

    The age and cigarette-smoking SMRs adjust for age and smoking differences between the industries' employees, using the indirect adjustment method.

    Because industries A and C show SMRs much higher than 100 (which are baseline standard for SMRs), some factors other than smoking and age are operative.

    Although the average annual death rate in B was high (71 per 100,000), adjustment for confounders of age and cigarette smoking shows its risk equal to industry E's and about equal to D's. Thus, cigarette smoking and age were related to lung cancer in B, which makes answer (b) incorrect.

8. Correct answer is (b). In the control table, it can be seen that there are differences in birthweights by class position in both rural and urban residents, but no real differences by places of residence in the two

classes. So when residence is controlled, only class is associated with birthweight.

9. a. Sensitivity is A/(A + C) so the correct answer is (3).
b. Specificity is D/(B + D) so (3) is the correct answer.
c. Frequency of false positives is B, so (2) is the correct answer.

10. If (a) is correct, you would need to find decline in incidence rates; if (b) is correct, a decline in case fatality ratios, suggesting improved treatment.

Table B.3   ***Incidence Rate and Case Fatality Ratio of Disease, by Year***

	Incidence rate	Case fatality ratio
1955	100/(50,000 − 100) = 2 per 1,000	5/200 = 25 per 1,000
1960	150/(75,000 − 75) = 2 per 1,000	5/225 = 22 per 1,000
1965	200/(100,000 − 50) = 2 per 1,000	5/250 = 20 per 1,000

Note: in calculating incidence rates, deduct cases that were *not* incidence cases from denominators in each year. These were probably from previous years and cannot be *new*. Because there is no secular change in incidence rates but a decline in case fatality ratios, (b) is the correct answer

11. a. (1) Is correct.
b. (2) Is correct.
c. (1) Is correct.

12. a. Correct answer is (1). Rare diseases are not easily studied in cohort style because we would need a large population to ascertain enough cases.
b. This needs a strategy to establish which precedes which. The best way is cohort; thus, correct answer is (2).
c. Selective survival does *not* bias the results of cohort studies, because we ascertain all of the cohort whether they survive or not. The correct answer is (1) case-control, for the cases studied and the controls are survivors; they may be selective in this.
d. Best quantification of attributable risk comes from cohort studies, thus, the answer is (2). Case-control studies can only *estimate* relative risk, at best.
e. Case-control (1).

Cohort studies over 20 years can be and have been done, but the logistics are very difficult and the low success rates in the continued participation and follow-up of participants make one not recommend it. An historical cohort is more advisable, but it was not given as an optional answer in this question.

13. The differences between 1937 and 1955 is that in 1937 there was no association with age of the death rates; in 1955, there was a possible association. No changes in the association with sex, males having higher rates than females at all ages.

a. Correct. The improvement of treatment over time among younger people would explain the positive association with age in 1955.

b. Correct. In 1955 doctors started labeling appendicitis deaths in younger people as something else, for example, alcoholic enteritis, which would artifactually reduce the rates in younger people; or doctors could have started increasing the labeling of deaths among older people as appendicitis in 1955. This would be a change in diagnostic custom.

c. Incorrect. The migration would have to be of young couples with *high* risk of death from appendicitis.

d. Incorrect. We are dealing with rates, so they are comparable.

14. Note that the prevalence in 1970 is higher in Framingham than in Puerto Rico—about twice as high. The incidence rate is five times as high in Framingham as in Puerto Rico in the ten-year period preceding 1970. Thus, if the death rates were the same in the two countries, one would expect the prevalence rate in Framingham to be about five times higher than in Puerto Rico. Since it is only 2.4 times higher, then the death rate in Framingham must be higher than in Puerto Rico. Thus (a) is correct. Immigration and cureism are not factors, as indicated.

15. a. This is incorrect—it is not relevant because indices are per capita or a proportion (a rate).

b. Unlikely explanation.

c. Correct. The investigator is using ecologic (group) indices and assuming associations, or lack thereof, between group indices.

d. Not correct—all are population-based.

16. Note in Table A.12 a positive association of distance and broken appointments. In Table A.13 the effect of social class has been nullified in the rates. The association found in Table A.12 is not seen in Table A.13. Therefore, social class must have been associated with distance, with the social class with greatest percentage of broken appointments also living further away.

a. Is correct. Because there is no association in Table A.13, the effect in Table A.12 must be social class dependent.
b. No, see (a).
c. Correct. See (a).
d. No. If that were so, Table A.13 would show some association.

17. Sensitivity speaks to likelihood of correctly identifying cases. Specificity speaks to likelihood of correctly identifying noncases.
a. This is concerned with having low rate of calling noncases sick (good specificity). Thus, pick B.
b. You overburden the health care system by having a high rate of false positives, that is, calling people as cases when they are not. So you want good calling of noncases, or specificity. Thus, pick B.
c. You need good case finding or sensitivity. Thus, pick A.
d. Same reasoning as in (c). Pick A.

18.

Table B.4   **Results of Two Observers'**
Independent Examinations for Diabetes (n = 100)

| | Observer A | | |
Observer B	Diabetics	Nondiabetics	Total
Diabetics	0	25	25
Nondiabetics	25	50	75
Total	25	75	100

19.

Table B.5   **Incidence and Prevalence Rates of**
Cancer in Children Aged 0-4, 1960–1970

Year	Incidence rates	Prevalence rates
1960	100/100,000 = 1/1,000	200/100,000 = 2/1,000
1965	120/150,000 = 0.8/1,000	350/150,000 = 2.3/1,000
1970	130/200,000 = 0.65/1,000	550/200,000 = 2.75/1,000

You would examine the new cases, as shown in Table B.5, and find that the incidence rate declines and the prevalence rate increases. Therefore, the preventive program is effective and treatment improving because prevalence is increasing. Correct answer is (c).

20. Note immediately that we are seeing data only on 136 cases of lead poisoning; there are no denominators at all.

Conclusion 1: Must be answer (b).
Conclusion 2: Clearly, admissions do occur more among summer months, so (c) must be correct. Bias due to seasonal variation in diagnostic custom can produce artifactual seasonal variations.

21. We would conclude that nonsmoking would save more workers from one disease than the other if attributable risks of death among smokers are different for the two diseases.

Attributable risk for lung cancer = 160-7 = 153/100,000

Attributable risk for CHD = 599-422 = 177/100,000
Therefore, (a) is incorrect; (b) is correct.

Relative risk for lung cancer = 160/7 = 23.7.

Relative risk for CHD = 599/422 = 1.4.
Therefore, (c) is correct; (d) is incorrect.

22. a. Incorrect. Age-specific rates in Table A.19 are *lower* in rural men, so different age distribution explains the higher total rate in rural men.
b. Correct.
c. Incorrect; rates are compared.
d. Incorrect; no bias was present.

23. For females, 80% of cases and 50% of controls (no accident) did not have driver education. For males, the rates are 40% and 40% respectively. Therefore:

a. (1) Incorrect. Conclusions are correct.
(2) Correct. Agree with conclusions, but they should have compared 80% with 50%; a "majority" of cases is not a comparison. They need to compare with noncases, where an equal "majority" may be found.
(3) Incorrect. The conclusions are correct.
(4) Incorrect. Did not make appropriate comparisons.

b. 40/50 and 50/100.
c. (1) Incorrect. Disagree with conclusions and the wrong comparisons were made.
(2) Incorrect. Disagree with conclusions.

(3) Correct.

(4) Disagree with conclusions.

d. 40/100, 80/200.

24. a. *If cross-sectional study:*

(1) True. Could have occurred.

(2) True.

(3) True. Higher case fatality rate in active men means few cases around in that group.

b. *If cohort study:*

(1) True.

(2) False. Persons classified on activity before occurrence of CHD.

(3) False. Case fatality ratio does not affect incidence rates.

References for Further Self-Evaluation Problems

This itemized list refers you to published available self-evaluation problems/exercises. The numbers listed are according to the main reference list at the end of this manual.

Reference number
4
16
20
25
27
29
40
46
47
53
60

Index

Page references to glossary entries are printed in **boldface** type.